LENAE GOOLSBY & TRIP GOOLSBY, MD

Think and Live Longer

Harnessing the secret laws of the universe for optimized health and longevity

Contents

The 7 Essential Life Spokes for Optimized Health & Life: Personal Assessment

To assess our achievements and progress, it can be beneficial to have a reference point. With that intention, LeNae presents this personal assessment.

This assessment is a mandatory exercise to begin the course and will serve as a starting point for the empowering journey you will embark on. We will revisit the assessment after completing the activities included in the following pages. The repetition of this assessment is important because it helps establish a mindset and create a successful health image, fostering a sense of fulfillment and accomplishment through periodic reviews.

Visual references provide guidance and help identify areas that require a shift in focus and energy. These visualizations highlight the various aspects and demands of our lives, as well as the impact they may have on our health. The periodic reviews allow us to evaluate and measure attributes, characteristics, habits, personal qualities, and empowering successes that we often overlook. These aspects far outweigh the adverse events that tend to dominate our attention. We create a healing environment by highlighting the gratitude we can cultivate in the face of significant health challenges and by promoting a higher energetic profile.

To complete the assessment, allocate fifteen to twenty minutes to reflect on different aspects of your life. You will better understand your current situation by rating yourself on a scale of one to ten for each category.

One signifies very poor, five represents a neutral state, and ten reflects a special status. Be honest with your ratings, as this exercise is for your benefit, and remember the phrase "To thine own self be true."

Once you have assigned ratings, divide each category by ten. For example, if your score under the "Family" category is 70, divide it by ten to obtain 7.0. Plot this value on the corresponding spoke for "Family." Repeat this process for all categories and connect the dots once all the values have been plotted. That's all there is to it! It's a straightforward exercise.

Spiritual

Belief in a divine creator ______
Faith ______
Intuitive ______
Sense of freedom to speak authentically ______
Inner peace ______
Compassion ______

Sense of personal power _______

Sense of personal creativity _______

Sense of feeling belongingness ____________

Total: Divided by 10 = ___________

Self-love

Daily fun activity ______

Fitness/exercise ______

Spend time with friends ______

Practice random acts of giving ______

Open to receiving ______

Spend time in meditation/reading ______

Practice prayer/gratitude ______

Spend time in personal development ______

Make nourishing choices ______

Other ______

Total: ___________

Total: Divided by 10 = ___________

Family

Strong family relationships ______

Feel respected _______

Feel accepted ______

Feel heard ______

Feel supported ______

Quality time together ______

Vacations ______

Constructively resolve differences ______

Affectionate ______

Other ______

Total: ___________

Total: Divided by 10 = ___________

Mental

Positive attitude ______
Logical/critical thinker ______
Creative/emotional ______
Strong formal education ______
Continuing education endeavors ________
Read Puzzles/games/brain exercises ______
Artistic/creative endeavors ______
Self-image ______
Other ______
Total: __________
Total: Divided by 10 = ___________

Physical Health

Happy with physical appearance ______
Strong energy and endurance ______
Positive results from regular checkups ______
Involved in an integrative health program ______
Pharmaceutical medication use for chronic medical problems*______
Engage in regular fitness activity ______
Healthy BMI ________
Good genes ________
Positive self-talk ________
Other ______
Total: ___________
Total: Divided by 10 = ___________

*For each chronic pharmaceutical medication used to manage

conditions such as blood pressure, blood sugar, cholesterol or lipids, pain, mood disorders, arthritis, and so on, deduct two points from the initial score of ten. It is important to note that the score can go into negative territory in this category.

Career

Love what you do ______

Exceed expectations ______

Positive colleague relationships ______

Feel like you fit with the team ______

Receive constructive feedback _______

Continuing training/education _______

Take leadership opportunities ______

Feel supported/valued _______

Aligned with company goals/vision/mission ______

Other ______

Total ___________

Total: Divided by 10 = ___________

Financial

Happy with income ______

Multiple revenue streams ______

Have clear financial goals and plan ______

Have and stay within budget ______

Have financial investments ______

Have savings account(s) ______

Have life/health insurance ______

Zero credit debt ______

Pay obligations on time ______

Other ______

Total ___________

Total: Divided by 10 = ______________

Great job! Now plot your results on the wheel to get the complete picture of your improvement opportunities!

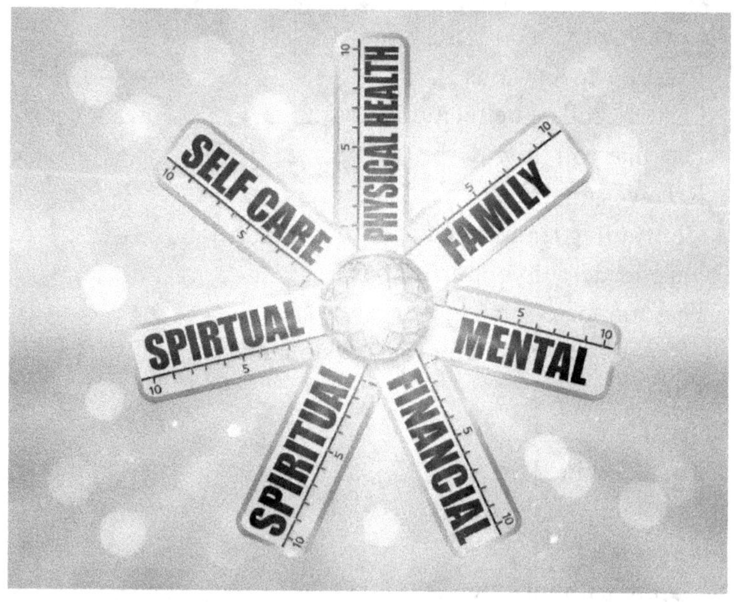

Preface

At the beginning of the twentieth century, William James, Ralph Waldo Emerson's godson, argued that individuals' inner attitudes can transform their outer lives. Despite such concepts in various historical writings, it is puzzling as to why it has taken us so long to integrate mind-body approaches into traditional medicine. Prescription drugs dominate our treatment strategies for illnesses, even though behavioral modifications can effectively address the same issues, often yielding superior results without unwanted side effects.

One explanation for this phenomenon is that physicians are trained to prescribe treatments based on peer-reviewed studies demonstrating positive outcomes with specific medical approaches, typically pharmaceutical or surgical. However, it is essential to recognize that researchers and participants in these studies impact the outcomes, contrary to the assumption of their impartiality.

This erroneous presumption has persisted since the early twentieth century. When we witness positive results from placebos or health-related affirmations, we must acknowledge the mind-over-health connection that manifests as inexplicable outcomes. We must question whether positive outcomes attributed to placebos result from misinterpreting the data or our misunderstanding of the actual effect. Can any positive outcome directly correlate with the participant's expectations—the "mind-body" effect?

Our beliefs and desires exert a profound influence on our health and well-being. In other words, we shape our health through our thoughts, ideas, actions, and habits as they interact with our genetic makeup. This phenomenon also explains, to a significant extent, the substantial differences in outcomes observed among individuals. I have witnessed these differential responses firsthand over many years of working with oncology patients at various disease stages and with integrative medicine patients with chronic diseases.

Is it simply a lack of awareness regarding our ability and power to contribute to a positive outcome that hinders our progress toward an empowering quantum medical approach?

Undoubtedly, this is a significant factor. Implementing a coherent, systematic approach that equips us with simple tools to motivate and empower behavioral change, delivered by compassionate and knowledgeable healthcare professionals, would significantly enhance our capacity to achieve desirable outcomes. As Gregg Braden, author of "The Spontaneous Healing of Belief," pointed out, *"The act of us simply looking at our world—projecting the feelings and beliefs that we have as we focus our awareness on the particles that the universe is made of—changes those particles as we are looking."*

Before proceeding, allow me to share more about my background.

In the autumn of 1975, I embarked on my journey to become a physician, following an unconventional path by learning French as a second language. Though unusual, this decision was prudent, given my family's expatriation to Belgium two years earlier because of my father's work with an international petroleum corporation. Being recognized as a Belgian national for educational purposes offered undeniable advantages.

After completing my studies at the Université Libre de Bruxelles, I completed an internal medicine internship and residency at the University of Health Sciences/Chicago Medical School, followed by a fellowship in oncology and hematology at Roswell Park Memorial Institute and the State University of New York at Buffalo.

Along the way, I had the incredible fortune of meeting the love of my life, LeNae. Our introduction occurred at a restaurant in Murfreesboro, Tennessee, in early 1998, facilitated by a mutual acquaintance. I remember feeling that a young woman of such extraordinary beauty could not possibly be interested in someone like me, a self-proclaimed geek. After a brief exchange of pleasantries, during which my ability to speak English coherently seemed to desert me, I swiftly escaped.

Given my social awkwardness at that first encounter, I was amazed when LeNae called my practice a few days later and asked if I would like to have dinner sometime to continue the scintillating conversation we had engaged in the previous evening. To this day – and my continued embarrassment – LeNae reminds me that my response to her invitation was an astonished laugh, followed by a fast, "Yes, I'd love to!"

After five years of dating and an equally clumsy proposal later, LeNae did me the incredible honor of becoming my wife. Before and after our marriage, our relationship has ushered several great perspectives and outcomes into my life. These miracles are the origin of a multitude of awakenings and enlightenments that informed this book and the methods I use to inspire, empower, and enhance my patients' health outcomes.

The first enlightenment I thought would not happen was the conception of our son, Henry IV. There were no issues with biology or chemistry, just my limiting belief that being a good father and the demands I imposed upon myself to provide the best outcomes for my patients were incompatible. I stopped believing this on the eve of my fiftieth birthday when Henry came into the world; four years later, Hayden Granger (aka Huckleberry) arrived.

> *"When the student is ready, the teacher will appear. When the student is truly ready... The teacher will disappear."* - Lao Tzu -Tao Te Ching

At that time, my interest in health optimization had peaked. I started investigating peer-reviewed therapeutic methods that could minimize the ravages of time on our physical bodies and perpetuate a dynamic health span.

This study led me to earn additional certifications and develop new practices, which I incorporated into my oncology practice. The successes my oncology patients achieved were quite impressive and gratifying, so I began expanding my integrative medicine practice using the techniques and data I had gathered. This was quite fortunate, as discord was brewing in my medical partnership. Putting my family above my affiliated nursing staff and colleagues caused conflict and catalyzed change. This shift in priority and awakened purpose provided insight into this book's transformative and motivational components.

My transformation and understanding came more from the personal effort and struggle resulting from my professional life change. I gained the perspective to recognize a body of motivational and transformational literature that has been the source of success for thousands—possibly millions—of individuals worldwide for millennia. This would lead to a profound epiphany. While devouring this literature, I noticed that these transformational methods were not being utilized specifically in the setting of disease management; it also occurred to me that the major chronic illnesses (those most effectively reversed by an optimized integrative approach, such as diabetes, cardiovascular disease, hypertension, depression, and anxiety, among others) were a ripe field for an empowerment approach that could motivate and assist in the transformation of lifestyle attitudes and habits that were the result of misinformation and/or limiting beliefs about our health.

In my imagination, I envisioned a form of "motivational medicine" or "transformational mindfulness" that could empower and uplift those who feel discouraged or defeated by conventional medicine. It is also for those who have become so accustomed to the current reactive, mass-produced healthcare system that they are unaware of their potential to create better health. This approach can complement treatments and increase the likelihood of a powerful mind-body response.

Around the same time, LeNae coincidentally enrolled in several intuitive empowerment training programs. As we discussed our respective journeys, we realized how interconnected they were. I immersed myself in the works of prominent thought leaders in the field of personal development, including Allen, Shinn, Hill, Proctor, Emerson, Byrne, Dyer, Hicks, Tolle, Singer, Vitale, Chopra, Dagher, Braden, Canfield, Ziglar, Murphy, Schucman, Thetford, Mundy, and others. Each page and every spoken word provided historical, philosophical, and religious insights that reached back to ancient times and encompassed a wide range of spiritual, religious, and metaphysical perspectives.

However, it was when I reviewed an online study course that LeNae took on Raymond Holliwell's work, offered by Bob Proctor and Mary Morrissey, that the idea of incorporating these teachings into a clinical process and writing this book took shape. I realized that the personal empowerment methods I had been studying aligned seamlessly with therapeutic imaging, biofeedback, and other current contemplative and mindfulness modalities. This empowered approach, which I have been implementing and documenting anecdotally, generates unprecedented compliance and enthusiasm for personal health and well-being transformation.

How can we best learn about and embrace the necessary changes to improve or eliminate harmful habits that contribute to poor health, limited longevity, and prolonged illness?

How can we overcome self-limiting beliefs, whether self-imposed or imposed by disillusioned healthcare providers, about achieving better health and longevity, regardless of the diagnosis?

What can we expect to achieve when implementing a motivational behavior modification program?

How can individuals who are not only burdened by disease but also by an impersonal, reactive healthcare system recognize that they have the power to achieve successful health outcomes?

I see universal laws as a mindful and transformational motivation to facilitate and enhance adherence to change. When understood and practiced, these laws enable us to respond constructively to the challenges we encounter in our daily lives. They provide confidence in our ability to create positive outcomes for ourselves and those around us.

Universal laws have a profound foundation across cultures, religions, and backgrounds, and their principles have captivated and motivated humanity throughout the ages. For example, in Christianity, there is the principle of sowing and reaping, where people harvest what they sow, emphasizing the importance of sowing positive things. In recent years, the Law of Attraction, which states that our thoughts, feelings, words, and actions attract energies of a similar nature, has gained popularity. While this law undoubtedly plays a crucial role in transforming our lives, it is not the sole principle at work. Different cultures recognize different numbers of universal laws, ranging from three to twelve or more. Regardless of the specific count, these laws are vital in helping us make the necessary changes to break free from harmful habits that contribute to the prevalence of chronic illnesses in our society. In this book, I have identified twelve laws for achieving optimal health, dedicating one chapter to each.

The realization that universal laws play a pivotal role in shaping our health, for better or worse, has been a profound revelation for my patients and me. Patients, counselors, and physicians can easily embrace these laws, enhancing personal determination, accountability, and discipline in adopting new behaviors and achieving improved outcomes for anyone willing to participate.

However, I firmly believe that the most effective approach is to combine the empowered and compassionate guidance of a "practitioner-coach." This practitioner-coach dynamic fosters the formation of intention, which combines belief, motivation, and resolve. It amplifies the potential for the quantum observer effect, in which observation changes the observed phenomenon. This applies to both the practitioner, who believes in the possibility of change and improvement, and the patient, who desires, believes, and intends to bring about change.

I gradually incorporated this empowered motivational training into my integrative medical practice alongside the medical and lifestyle methods we employ. Our core 4-Pillar Approach to health optimization encompasses transformational mind-body practices, nutritional optimization, physical optimization, and the integration of bio-identical hormones and metabolic optimization. This approach significantly improves the quality of life. It enables most of my patients to reduce or eliminate their dependence on prescription medications for chronic diseases such as diabetes, hypertension, depression, and chronic anxiety.

This integrative medical practice eventually led to the founding of the Infinite Health Integrative Medical Center, which now offers a range of services (for more information, visit www.YourInfiniteHealth.com). When patients are empowered to become creators of their health, they can actively improve their attitudes, perspectives, and lives while eliminating the need for toxic pharmaceutical medications. Compliance with lifestyle measures is enhanced by motivational and transformational contemplative practices, complemented by bioidentical hormone optimization and metabolic correction to address underlying imbalances.

Empowered motivation alleviates anxiety, reduces failure, and promotes adherence in anyone striving for better health. The application of universal laws tailored to each patient's unique medical situation follows a logical sequence that can be consciously applied to health-related challenges and other aspects of life that commonly coexist.

By adopting this approach, we can effectively address individual compliance weaknesses and resolve issues that often lead to failure when similar approaches are absent. The simple incorporation of daily mindfulness and contemplative imaging techniques makes it easier to achieve these changes. While the examples provided here may reflect a single-institution and investigator bias, I am confident that individuals seeking real, effective life changes for better health can be empowered and transformed through this methodology. LeNae and I have written this book to help people understand and embrace this approach, empowering them to achieve the healing and long-lasting quality of life we all deserve.

—Trip Goolsby, MD

Introduction

*"The greatest revolution of our generation is the
discovery that human beings,
by changing the inner attitudes of their minds,
can change the outer aspects of their lives."*

This quote, often attributed to William James and Albert Schweitzer, emphasizes the power of an empowered mind-body approach in various aspects of our lives, not just physical health. It also reflects the author's desire to share practical wisdom with those who could greatly benefit from this empowering perspective. Let's consider ourselves energetic spiritual beings undergoing a physical experience and understand that one of our purposes in this embodiment is to advance and learn. We should have the opportunity and information necessary to do so. And indeed, these opportunities for growth and learning present themselves in various ways, whether sought out through our curiosity or imposed upon us. They arise precisely when we need them.

However, many challenges and efforts required to succeed

in any therapeutic plan demand significant motivation and dedication. Complex, multiple disease processes require even greater energy and motivation from the affected individual to achieve successful recovery. The motivational awareness and mindfulness techniques presented in the following chapters aim to help each person create their desired state of thriving health.

The pursuit of knowledge is intrinsically linked to the need for knowledge, whether or not an individual recognizes that need. Often, we stumble or fall (sometimes quite literally) as we pass through the gate of learning. A perfect example is a broken hip resulting from osteoporosis, which frequently occurs due to prolonged hormonal and vitamin deficiencies associated with aging.

Another example is the onset of diabetes, the culmination of hormonal imbalances, diminishing insulin levels, poor dietary habits, and often long-standing obesity, rendering insulin ineffective in blood sugar control. These examples demonstrate how the need for knowledge remains unknown until our youthful reserves are depleted, mainly, and disease symptoms manifest suddenly in our lives. Then we realize the need for information and turn to sources like Google to acquire knowledge that mirrors our physicians'. Often, we discover that our conditions are not sudden at all but the result of lifestyle habits adopted over time, which are often of questionable benefit or outright detrimental.

In *"Think and Live Longer,"* we have distilled a template of empowerment, a pathway many of our patients have successfully followed to achieve various health goals. We intend to provide a clear understanding of the concepts that our patients have questioned throughout their journeys. In my practice, much time is spent interpreting the practical implications of universal laws within the context of individual patient challenges. In this book, we explain these laws so that you can gain a practical ability to apply them to your medical issues and integrate them into your pursuit of optimized health. More than physical examinations or the review of lab and imaging results, embracing the concepts of personal health creation has been the true turning point for most of my patients. Achieving success in long-term health optimization becomes more accessible when clear guidelines are established, and a vivid image of the desired outcome is formed.

The concepts of universal laws presented here are often intuitively understood by many people, even if they are unaware of their importance or implications. When these laws are consciously integrated into daily thoughts, behaviors, and habits, they promote objective Awareness of challenges that may otherwise trigger adverse bodily responses and exacerbate chronic diseases. Unaware of the impact of these laws, we need help creating the desired experiences throughout our lifetime, not only in terms of lifestyle desires but also in optimizing our health and well-being. Developing a clear understanding and concept in our minds is one of the most empowering exercises we can undertake.

In the words of Dr. Deepak Chopra, *"Everything that exists in the physical world is the result of the un-manifest transforming itself into the manifest ... anything and everything that we can perceive through our senses—is the transformation of the un-manifest, unknown and invisible into the manifest, known, and visible."* This aligns with the idea that we continually shape our bodies through the environment we create internally, influenced by nutrition, exposures, and our responses to external stimuli and experiences. These internal responses either support our healing and well-being or contribute to illness. They also serve as a source of empowerment, enabling us to achieve our health goals.

The rationale behind the treatments and lifestyle changes many of us must adopt to succeed in health optimization rests on two main factors: genetic blueprints and functional reserve. We inherit genetic blueprints (DNA) from our parents, which serve as templates for our lives, health, and well-being. If we respect these blueprints and avoid abusing them, we maintain better health and well-being for longer. Conversely, if we consistently disregard them, we will face the consequences of our actions.

Understanding the components of health outcomes is crucial for individuals and the health insurance industry. The data indicate that only 10% of healthcare outcomes are directly related to medical care, while 30% are attributed to our underlying genetic makeup (genome). The remaining sixty percent is influenced by individual behavior and social and environmental factors (forty percent and twenty percent, respectively). Additionally, a study in 2006 by J. Hjelmborg and colleagues revealed that genetic makeup only accounted for ten to twenty-five percent of longevity, with the remaining seventy-five to ninety percent attributed to lifestyle choices.

Medical research in basic and clinical neuroscience is advancing rapidly, demonstrating how our thoughts influence the mapping of pathways to achieve our desired goals, including optimizing our health. While these concepts are gaining recognition within the theoretical knowledge base of medicine, there remains a need to qualify and implement them in practical ways to effectively support individuals. In my integrative medical practice, I have found that a step-wise approach involving exercises and studying these laws has been highly effective, benefiting not only those with multiple health challenges but also individuals who are gradually depleting their health reserves.

Why don't we feel as well as we did in earlier stages of life? It's not solely due to aging. Time certainly plays a role in the evolution of our well-being, but our choices determine the outcomes we desire, whether passively or actively. As Ralph Waldo Emerson noted in his discourse on compensation, "*A perfect equity adjusts its balance in all parts of life. 'Oi chusoi Dios aei enpiptousi!' The dice of God are always loaded.*" For human beings, the balance of outcomes allows us to improve our health and longevity by sowing the right seeds. As Mr. Emerson astutely observed, we will always be compensated for our lives and choices (or avoid making). Our organs possess an impressive "functional reserve," meaning we can eliminate up to 80% or more of an organ's function without endangering our survival. We can continue to thrive, improve, and perform relatively well. However, if we eliminate a few more percentage points from this marginal function, symptoms, malaise, illness, and disease emerge, accompanied by a loss of the invulnerability we felt in our youth.

When faced with these sudden circumstances, we try to recapture the vigor of our youth by increasing exercise duration, changing our diet, and increasingly turning to multiple supplements and nutraceuticals (nutrients with claimed or proven results that don't require a prescription). The burning question in our minds is, *"What can enhance my declining stamina and sense of well-being and take me back to the 'glory days'?"* Integrative physicians typically offer corrective lifestyle changes as the first step, followed by medication if necessary. However, we must also answer the accompanying question, *"What am I willing to change to achieve that?"* In answering this question, the insights and motivation provided by this book become most valuable.

By becoming more mindful of how we cultivate discipline and motivation, we give ourselves the fuel needed for change. This fuel has helped not only those seeking recovery from serious diseases but also those focused on slowing or preventing morbidity and decline. We now understand that subtle changes in multiple laboratory parameters are associated with a silent yet clinically meaningful decline in longevity and quality of life as we age. Armed with this knowledge, we have the power to effect change.

Most of the healthier parameters resemble those from our younger years. For example, maintaining certain hormone levels in the upper 20% of our lifetime values reduces the risk of heart attack and stroke. Optimization also significantly improves our well-being and sustains a biologically youthful vascular infrastructure.

The information that governs our reserve is inherited from our parents and encoded in our DNA. DNA consists of numerous proteins and enzymes and forms twenty-three pairs of chromosomes. The Human Genome Project, completed in 2001, identified approximately 23,000 genes in the human genome. Through transcription, these genes give rise to an unknown number of proteins (the proteome). Estimates suggest that between 150,000 and two million proteins may be formed and incorporated into the human body. How is this possible? How can twenty-three thousand genes produce such a vast array of proteins? The answer lies in the fact that our genome can be interpreted and expressed through a complex system of reactions known as epigenetics. This is where I would like to introduce EVE: the Epigenetic Variability Effector.

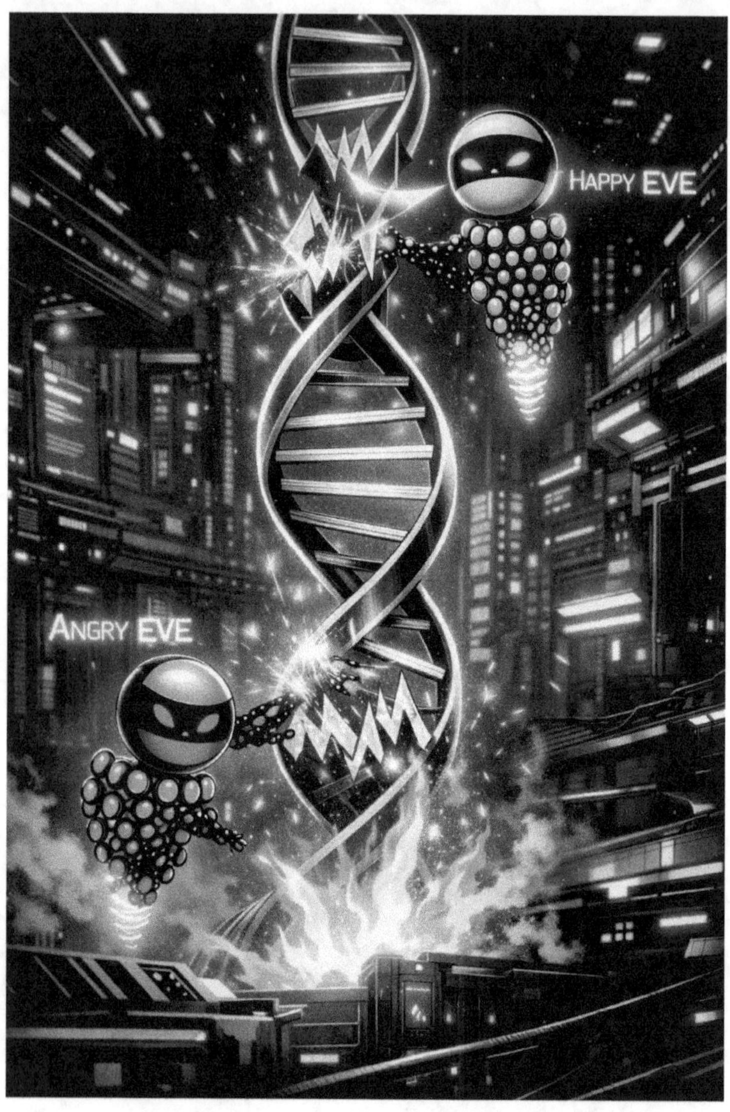

EVE represents my personalized concept of an intelligent integration of molecular biological activities that can either enhance, maintain, or compromise cellular function based on the information it receives. Each cell in our body has its own epigenetic infrastructure that interprets and guides subsequent biomolecular events, determining whether DNA expression and interpretation are positive or negative. In simpler terms, EVE can respond positively, negatively, or neutrally to external stimuli such as food, toxins, radiation, and other factors, as well as internal factors like metabolic and hormonal changes influenced by our interactions with the world and our thoughts. These responses can affect the cell's outcome and survival, and ultimately the individual's survival. Some of these changes are transient, lasting only a few cell cycles.

In contrast, others can be imprinted for a lifetime and even passed on to future generations, even without the initial transformative exposure.

The information that triggers epigenetic modifications can originate from within the body or from external sources. The effects of external information are relatively easy to grasp and encompass various factors such as nutrition, pharmaceuticals, physical agents, infections, and toxins, all of which can potentially influence our epigenome. The emerging field of nutritional epigenomics, for instance, explores how the elemental composition of food affects DNA expression and how this, in turn, leads to pathways that promote individual well-being. This suggests that in the near future, we may be able to select meals that specifically modulate different aspects of our genome.

The influence of internal information primarily stems from our hormonal and autonomic nervous systems, and from how their actions affect the organs essential for sustaining life. Chapter two further delves into this system, emphasizing its crucial significance and providing exercises to engage with it. The cumulative effects of these epigenetic modifications create an environment that either depletes, disregards, or enhances the reserves of our various organ systems.

By reading and engaging with the exercises in this book, we develop the ability to focus on desired outcomes and the means to achieve them. It becomes a tool that empowers us to not only attain the desired level of health but also to activate our imagination and beliefs to manifest an environment and circumstances that align with our vision of successful health. It represents an affirmative, mindful, and complementary step towards self-realized health, healing, and well-being. It utilizes empowered awareness to cultivate a lasting quality of life and the healing of illness we all deserve.

The Infinite Law of Success in Health

*"If we did all the things we are capable of doing,
we would literally astound ourselves."* —Thomas A.
Edison

I first encountered Fran* several days after she was admitted to the hospital due to septic shock. This life-threatening bacterial infection can cause heart failure and a severe drop in blood pressure. Before this critical health crisis, Fran, a seventy-eight-year-old woman, had been dealing with multiple medical issues that significantly impacted her quality of life. These included severe obesity and adult-onset diabetes with complications such as nerve damage, kidney damage, eye damage, vascular disease, and coronary artery disease. According to her latest echocardiogram, she had also undergone a triple bypass surgery a few years earlier and had congestive heart failure according to her latest echocardiogram. Additionally, Fran had chronic obstructive pulmonary disease (COPD), degenerative arthritis in her lower back and knees, gout, and rheumatoid arthritis.

Fran was transferred to my care from a nearby community

when her compromised kidney function and heart failure led to the buildup of chemotherapy drugs in her body, resulting in bone marrow failure and the depletion of white blood cells (which protect against infections) and platelets (cells that help stop bleeding). Remarkably, with the efforts of my colleagues and me, we were able to restore her marrow function by administering medications to stimulate the production of new white blood cells and providing transfusions of red blood cells and platelets. Throughout this process, she received high doses of antibiotics and antifungal medications that became necessary.

About eight days after her admission, when Fran no longer required ventilator support or blood pressure assistance, she could finally communicate with me for the first time. Her recovery was slow, initially in the hospital and later at home, taking four to six weeks.

During her outpatient visit, Fran appeared remarkably frail and relied on a wheelchair for mobility. She depended on her three daughters, who lived nearby, for assistance. However, she maintained her mental clarity and expressed a genuine desire to regain as much of her previous physical function as possible, if not surpass it. Fran had been an avid gardener in her healthier days and wished to return to that activity or achieve something even better, something she hadn't been able to enjoy for the past two to three years.

Over the following ten months, we collaborated using a comprehensive approach that optimized nutrition, exercise, and endocrine/metabolic factors. Fran followed a low-carbohydrate diet, which reduced her dependency on insulin and allowed me to decrease her oral medications for blood sugar control from three to one. As Fran was postmenopausal, I prescribed bioidentical hormone replacement therapy and optimized her thyroid and adrenal hormones.

However, Fran's family members, specifically her two daughters, expressed concern about my recommended approach. They believed that Fran's multiple health conditions restricted her ability to engage in any physical activity beyond the most limited level. They opposed the idea of gardening or using aerobic exercise equipment, fearing that it would cause pain due to her arthritis and potentially trigger a heart attack. They also objected to using additional hormones, wrongly assuming it would lead to complications.

The intensity of their reaction made me feel as if two of Fran's daughters might metaphorically "lynch" me before the day was over. Nonetheless, I stood my ground, emphasizing that improving Fran's overall condition would require incremental efforts across nutritional, nutraceutical, and hormonal interventions. Fran's vision of success was to surpass her pre-hospitalization state, and I was determined to facilitate that goal as long as it didn't jeopardize my own life. If it hadn't been for the intervention of the eldest daughter, who diffused the situation, I might not have survived to write this account.

Fran, who had listened intently as I explained the plan and the rationale, was all in. Her vision of success was clear. She provided the effort and forgave the two younger daughters' limited beliefs in her abilities. She worked at her maximum capacity at all times; her successful health image was one of independence in the home, walking to the daughters' houses in reasonably close proximity, and planting and managing the garden of her dreams again without assistance.

A year after Fran's hospitalization, she walked into my office with the aid of only a cane. She frequently walked to her daughters' houses nearby and gardened as she saw fit, to the amazement—and appreciation—of the two daughters. Given the nature of her accomplishments, I was also curious to assess her cardiopulmonary recovery, as she was no longer short of breath when walking. I suggested we obtain a follow-up echocardiogram to assess her left ventricular ejection fraction (a measure of heart function). The results were incredible! New tests showed an impressive 38%, up considerably from the 18% indicated by hospital testing. She also experienced many other functional improvements, which accompanied a significantly improved quality of life, and she continued to improve further after that. The number of different medications for blood pressure and arthritis was also reduced and/or discontinued during the same period.

Fran remains one of the most poignant examples of how much we can accomplish in the face of devastating, debilitating chronic disease when we focus on a specific vision of health success. This is a simple case, but it illustrates what an optimized integrative approach can achieve.

We are all created capable of having the health we desire in that we live, for the most part, for years and years without the slightest hint of encumbrance. This grace period largely depends on the genetic gifts our parents pass down to us (our genome). That genome determines the sensitivity of our reserve to the lifestyle we subject it to. As we subject our genome to our daily lifestyle trauma, its reserve, and our end organs are consumed. Finally, when we have exhausted most or all of the reserves we were gifted with at birth, we develop symptoms and signs of disease. But this is not the end. Even when disease (dis-ease) becomes apparent, we may regain a significant degree of our health, if not all, by committing to a guided recovery program. Most of us want to do just that upon receiving this wake-up call. It is a critical turning point that allows us to change direction, and the extent of our recovery depends on the image we choose to focus on.

Those of us who understand the nature of this underlying reserve and/or are fortunate enough to work with a practitioner who is prepared to assist in optimizing the reserve, instead of simply giving yet another pill, can, to the degree their reserve permits, become the masters of their future health outcome

How do we know what that reserve is?

While numerous studies enable physicians to assess when an organ is likely to fail and require artificial support (dialysis, mechanical ventilation, etc.), there are currently no reliable means to predict how much we can recuperate by optimizing residual reserve. Nor can we determine the point at which damage incurred over a lifetime precludes any recovery, if this point exists at all. There are several hypotheses, but they have not yet been verified and would be highly individual and case-specific, related to the individual's genomic and end-organ reserve. One would hope that this information, when acquired, would come from studies that reflect a quantum perspective in both their design and interpretation. This will be clarified in the years to come.

We know we are born with incredible resilience and flexibility in recovering from injury and other insults. The plasticity of the different organ systems and their ability to recover is inborn and always ready to respond, adapt, and help us recover from even the most catastrophic events. Many individuals in our optimization programs know this and make full use of its recovery potential. The treatment programs in our practice are individually tailored to each patient based on their unique parameters and medical challenges. Our personalized mind-body approach is also tailored to each patient's specific challenges and woven into the foundation of the universal laws coaching format. It is adapted dynamically based on the individual, their responses, and situational challenges throughout clinical improvement and optimization.

Each of us has the potential for seemingly endless improvement in any aspect of our lives. This ability is a natural creative process defined and embedded in our genetic makeup. Understanding the nature of this self-empowering gift gives us the robust ability to succeed in any convalescence (or any other endeavor) we choose. I allude to the simple effect we see in athletic circles about record-setting performances. Regardless of the level an athlete attains, numerous studies will always help them create and achieve the right, successful image.

Some may think your ability to recover or improve is beyond

your physical capacity. I can assure you that you will be reflecting, as Mr. Edison did in the opening statement: *"If we did all the things we are capable of doing, we would literally astound ourselves."* But, in order to achieve this, you must follow your earnest desires and use the universal laws to embolden your behavior and connect yourself to the source of all that becomes real and tangible in your existence. In so doing, you become the empowered creator of your health reality.

If nature—the universe—is ignorant of failure, it is because s/he recognizes that **all the natural universal laws are always working together to enhance our health**. What does this mean? Think about the seed that grows into a tree or the broken bone that begins to heal as soon as the fracture has occurred. Healing events are assured and occur without fail. This happens because all laws governing the reactions that lead to recovery or growth are satisfied.

Furthermore, when we are simultaneously in harmony with these natural or universal laws, we become an indistinguishable force of creation. With that empowerment, we should understand that we are never limited in our abilities to recover, improve, and develop our health. No matter where we are when we begin, we will reap a successful outcome! Recent research on how our internal and external environments influence our body's genetic makeup supports this statement. Based on the environment that bathes our cells, these epigenetic changes can, if you will, regenerate our body over time. The results of this cellular regeneration will be accomplished to our benefit - or our detriment - depending on how we create this environment. At every moment, our choice should be to create nurturing, supportive surroundings that allow our cells to thrive!

When we understand and collectively apply the universal laws, the probability of success increases significantly. Why is this? Unlike the successful business executive or professional, we are better served - and have fewer chances of failure - if we have **guidelines by which a successful outcome might be obtained.** Learning, adapting to, and adhering to these laws gives us awareness, perspective, tempered knowledge, and the thoughtful ability to work harmoniously with the forces of universal good and creation. This awareness and our commitment to a new affirmative behavioral foundation, in concert with these laws, allow us to nurture, grow, and advance. It is a process of establishing a correct understanding of the principles upon which constructive, successful achievement might be founded. These achievements will, in turn, lead to the healthier, longer lifestyle—what I like to call the "health span"—that we desire.

What does success mean?

Success is the favorable, prosperous culmination of our endeavors or goals. However, the definition of success is subjective and varies based on an individual's beliefs and perspective. It also depends on whether the person considers their efforts to pursue a goal complete.

The Universal Law of Success assures us that we have unlimited resources available to accomplish any goal we undertake. It confirms that we possess the necessary infrastructure to embark on a regenerative health journey or any other endeavor we choose. With this understanding, it becomes clear that we can achieve whatever goals we set for ourselves.

The question then arises: What does success mean to you?

"What is success? To laugh often and much; To win the respect of intelligent people and the affection of children; To earn the appreciation of honest critics and endure the betrayal of false friends; To appreciate beauty; To find the best in others; To leave the world a bit better, whether by a healthy child, a garden patch or a redeemed social condition; To know even one life has breathed easier because you have lived; This is to have succeeded." —Ralph Waldo Emerson

This understanding should come to us due to our logical, cognitive, and intuitive abilities. What I frequently see, however, is that we sell ourselves short because we lack an understanding of what we can achieve. Many reasons for these limiting beliefs become clinically and glaringly apparent during my patients' initial visits. Sadly, the most frequent cause is that a limiting belief has been imposed upon an individual by their treating physician. How many times have I heard, *"Several doctors have told me that I will never do* (fill in the blank) *again,"* or *"This will never get any better,"* or *"I will just have to live with it"*? This is a form of limiting belief imposed upon us by others that we have accepted as unconditional truth. When applied to our lives (the life of a single individual, not the estimated average of a species), however, these limiting beliefs are invariably hypothetical, unsubstantiated, and ultimately untrue. On the other hand, **when we affirm our ability to succeed by desire and heartfelt intuition our ability to succeed, we also invariably set and subsequently attain our goals!**

"The indispensable first step to getting the things you want out of life is this: Decide what you want." —Ben Stein

Once we have established our healthcare goal, we must put in the effort to achieve it. Our desire is like the gas that powers the engine of progress, driving us forward; it generates the initiative to build new foundations of personal preparedness and capability.

We can all develop our hidden talents, intellect, intuition, and hidden and unknown strengths in pursuing the health-related goals we desire to achieve. Vision and intention are the keys that will provide access to the energy of desire. They are the universal resources that subsidize success. And that success is valid for any health-related desire we so choose.

No person can succeed who is not imbued with the desire to advance ... The desire to advance implies the power to advance ... The fact that you desire to succeed is evidence that you have the power to succeed; otherwise, you would not have been urged to aspire success-ward. — Raymond Holliwell, author of Working with the Law:

11 Truth Principles for Successful Living

Whether discussing healthcare or any other aspect of life, continued progress toward our goals is the yardstick for defining success or impending failure. Failure, by definition, occurs only when we have terminated all effort that defines forward progress; acceptance of the challenge of temporary failure, however, is moving toward the established goal. This means that, while en route to the health we wish to achieve, we may need to learn new things; for example, conducting an Internet search on things that will help us achieve our happy end result.

We also may need to establish a new plan for an advance after a setback. If necessary, we regroup with our Medical Mastermind, the group of mentors, motivators, and healthcare providers who work harmoniously at our behest to promote our successful health image. This asset has an exponential probability of resolving our challenges and further strengthening our determination to move forward.

Setting small goals that draw us ever closer to the final one is another critical approach, particularly for those dealing with longstanding chronic health problems. Doing so enables us to celebrate intermediate successes as we assimilate changes in small bites. Setting small goals also allows for smaller setbacks if there is a minor failure; the "indigestion" (frustration) will be more tolerable along the way.

If you want to be happy, set a goal that commands your thoughts,
liberates your energy, and inspires your hopes.
—Andrew Carnegie

The Law of Success is characterized by an unstoppable forward momentum, much like the laws of nature. Our ability to envision success in terms of our health determines what we can achieve (which will be further emphasized in the Law of Supply).

We should never fear the most excellent possible outcome we can intuitively create because that is precisely what we can actualize in the future. This is possible because we have the innate capacity to learn, create, and improve ourselves to attain any physical, emotional, and mental state we can imagine. Furthermore, when our intuition guides us, we constantly communicate with infinite intelligence (or a higher power). The empowering desires in our hearts are bestowed upon us because we can accomplish them. We are also always connected to the resources required to bring our imaginations to life, including our health.

If we intuitively imagine achieving a health goal, we can not only achieve it but also surpass it. Proverbs 4:23 states, *"Guard your heart above all else, for everything you do flows from it."* This suggests that success is assured if we sincerely establish our goals and action plans with sincerity and ensure that our thoughts and subsequent actions align with our integrity and purpose. However, obstacles may arise along our journey, particularly if we deviate from the principles that help us maintain focus on our goals.

Fear of failure or success is a dangerous obstacle we must not allow into our consciousness. And why should we? When infinite intelligence has provided us with the vision of success, no obstacle can ultimately thwart it. The following poem by Guillaume Apollinaire often reflects my interactions with my patients, who may need more information or have experienced numerous setbacks or failures. Unfortunately, being a patient in a conventional reactive care setting often diminishes their initiative, desire, and intention to achieve better outcomes. However, it is remarkable how well the laws of success support and empower these individuals as they embrace a new approach and step outside the confines of conventions.

Take a Leap of Faith and Fly!
"Come to the edge," he said.
We can't, we're afraid," they responded.
"Come to the edge," he said.
And so they came.
And he pushed them.
And they flew.

There exists a great reservoir of untapped potential for good health, even in individuals who are severely ill. This has been repeatedly demonstrated in numerous clinical cases. For example, consider the stories of individuals paralyzed after strokes who go on to recover and lead normal lives or athletes who are told they will never compete again but miraculously return and win. Even Fran's story defies conventional thinking and expectations, and I must admit that in the first few months after her discharge, my own belief wavered at times. The fact that such a reservoir of potential exists enables and empowers the desire to achieve. It ignites an insatiable hunger for success, to the extent that we only need to think, speak, and act as if we already possess it for it to become a reality (see the law of supply).

Believe and behave as if failure were impossible.
—Charles F. Kettering

I am constantly amazed by the correlation between individuals' outward demeanor when facing health challenges and the outcomes they achieve. The final results I have observed are undeniably linked to individual patients' thoughts, attitudes, and beliefs, particularly their vision of successful health. The most crucial attitude for success is believing in *"I can!"* This mindset often leads to positive outcomes by instilling the desire and initiative needed to overcome both major and minor obstacles along the path to the desired goal. The momentum generated by *"I can!"* fulfills the promise of inspiration and empowered creativity. Affirming *"I can!"* helps generate the ideas needed to overcome the roadblocks that frequently impede our progress toward success.

"Nothing can stop the man with the right mental

attitude from achieving his goal; nothing on earth can help the man with the wrong mental attitude."
—Thomas Jefferson

Those who lead a lifestyle that has led to chronic disease and endangers their lives do not have to remain bound to that lifestyle until their demise. We should not believe that change is impossible or that we cannot succeed because we have always done things a certain way. Each of us is an incredible, infinite being endowed with the ability to assess challenges and change our unhealthy behaviors. Every person's brain possesses that capacity; we need only embrace the power of the two simple words: "I can!" These words empower us to cultivate desire and the momentum for change to achieve our desired health. Therefore, we can all achieve success in our health, regardless of the specific goals we choose.

Thinking

by Walter D. Winkle

If you think you are beaten, you are,
If you think you dare not, you don't,
If you'd like to win, but think you can't
It's almost a cinch, you won't
If you think you'll lose, you're lost,
For out in the world we find,
Success begins with a fellow's will
It's all in the state of mind.
If you think you're outclassed, you are,
You've got to think high to rise.

You've got to be sure of yourself before
You can ever win a prize.
Life's battles don't always go
To the stronger or faster man,
But soon or late the man who wins
Is the man WHO THINKS HE CAN!

We assess our patient-partner applicants to determine their level of desire and attitude. Interestingly, many patients who initially believe they cannot succeed when coached on the implications of the negative attitude can shift into a can-do attitude and succeed over time. This depends, of course, on the desire for a positive outcome. As with attitude, we gauge desire and motivation on a simple one-to-ten subjective scale. We also inform patients that the phrase "I can't!" is considered a vulgarity and must be eliminated from their vocabulary, particularly during their initial training.

The phrase *"I can!"* is crucial in the mind-body program. It generates an empowering, positive attitude that is evident in the words themselves. When we engage our affirmative ability to take action related to our health, our creativity and determination are enhanced, enabling us to formulate a path toward achieving our imagined goal. In that affirmation, we envision the victorious conqueror who assembles and summons all the necessary resources and relationships to thrive.

"In all circumstances, you are greater than the things or
the conditions; if not actually, you are

potentially... Whatever you lack, He has; whatever you need, He can supply; whatever obstacle you encounter, God within you and about you can overcome it." - Raymond Holliwell

* * *

The Think and Live Longer Mind Shift Hack: Visualize Your Successful Health Image

This exercise is designed to help you establish the parameters of your success and improve your well-being. The image you create will act as an anchor, connecting you to your desired outcome. The more detailed your image, the easier it becomes to measure your progress. You can celebrate your successes more readily when you achieve the description you create here and emotionally relate to it.

It is also suggested that the image and its surroundings, including objects, locations, and people, should evoke a sense of gratitude or happiness. Joy and gratitude have healing vibrations that promote relaxation and peacefulness, which can help resolve or manage chronic diseases such as high blood pressure and diabetes.

To begin, conceptualize and write down at least twenty different health characteristics that describe your ideal optimized healthy image. While creating this list, you may find it helpful to surround yourself with objects, people, locations, events, and activities that enhance your image and evoke feelings of success.

Sometimes this exercise can be challenging for individuals, so additional guidelines are provided to assist with the imaging process. One helpful approach is to subject the creative image to specific criteria. The most effective criteria we have found are FORM, FEELING, and FUNCTION, which empower and guide individuals in creating their ideal optimized health image.

FORM is the external appearance that best represents our empowered, healthy image. It should be clearly defined by measurable metrics that define optimum health and bodily dimensions. For example, we should not settle for a physical appearance that perpetuates poor health and chronic disease. Population-based data suggest that minimizing total body fat to 18% for women and 15% for men optimizes potential health span and longevity. To help patients understand this aspect, I often use the analogy of time travel. I suggest imagining they have reached a future point where they have achieved their ideal Successful Health Image (SHI). They can then meet their new SHI, which will briefly and affirmatively describe itself using the appropriate metrics.

FEELING is the second factor that requires attention, as many of us have adapted to compromises and restrictions in our lifestyles. We are like frogs in hot water, where gradual heating allows us to remain unaware of the need to escape. But if we are suddenly dropped into preheated water, we immediately react to avoid harm. Similarly, we may have incredible reserves, but the progressive restrictions we impose on ourselves are compromises that an optimized integrative approach can recover if the image is correct. Focusing on the sense of well-being we experienced as teenagers or young adults can help us find the descriptive vocabulary for the optimized health image we seek.

Lastly, the FUNCTION of our diverse organs is critical to our overall well-being and our ability to engage in daily activities. Mental and cognitive functions, sensory functions, cardiorespiratory, digestive, kidney, hematologic, immune, and musculoskeletal functions all play vital roles. Describing the optimal capabilities of these functions in the SHI helps optimize the process.

Take a few moments to relax, close your eyes, and visualize your optimized health and lifestyle. This is just the first step in achieving your empowered health outcome. When you feel ready, complete the exercise using the provided form. Be mindful of using affirmative statements and avoid negative terms such as "no," "not," "without," "don't," and so on.

These statements should be brief, in the present tense, and assert your affirmations in the first person.

For example: "I am ___________," "I ___________ daily," "I have ___________," "I ___________," "I love to ___________," and so on.

Lastly, objective measurements help establish a quantitative endpoint that allows for celebrations of success. For example, if you can run a mile in seven minutes, that becomes a measurable benchmark. In the FORM section, consider how all aspects of your new body look, focusing on numbers, sizes, and dimensions as essential qualifiers.

FORM (Physical Appearance)	Example: My body is strong	Example: I move gracefully

FEELING (How do I feel about myself and how I interact with the world around me?)

FEELING (Emotion)	Example: I feel confident	Example: I love all aspects of my body.

FUNCTION (How do my body and organs work for me in my new Successful Health Image?)

FUNCTION (What you can do)	Example: I run a mile in 8 minutes	Example: I practice meditation and do yoga daily.
	47	

The Infinite Law of Thinking in Health

*All that we are is the result of what we have thought; it
is founded on our thoughts; it is made up of our
thoughts.*—Buddha

Gregg was an intriguing patient who, according to his admission, remained oblivious to his role in developing his multiple chronic health issues. His upbringing by his mother, who constantly labeled him as the "sickly sibling," profoundly impacted his mindset. He frequently referred to these experiences when discussing his ailments, firmly stating, *"That's how I've always been, and that's how I'll always be. It's not my fault!"*

Unfortunately, Gregg missed a follow-up appointment because he was admitted to the hospital due to acute pancreatitis, a potentially life-threatening inflammation of the pancreas. His symptoms included nausea, vomiting, severe abdominal pain, and jaundice. He underwent surgery to remove his gallbladder, which contained gallstones that had caused a blockage in his common bile duct, resulting in an episode of acute pancreatitis.

Upon returning for a check-up three weeks later, Gregg said, *"I had nothing to do with it."* However, the truth was that Gregg had several health conditions and lifestyle choices that predisposed him to gallstones and triggered the subsequent pancreatitis attack. These conditions were primarily associated with his morbid obesity, adult-onset diabetes, a diet high in carbohydrates (sugars), and a lack of fiber. He also had hyperlipidemia, a condition characterized by elevated levels of various fats in the blood, and hypercholesterolemia, excessive cholesterol in the bloodstream, which had not been adequately addressed despite using cholesterol-lowering medications (another risk factor for gallstones). In addition, Gregg experienced hypogonadism (undetected and untreated low levels of sexual hormones), hypertension, suboptimally treated hypothyroidism (insufficient thyroid hormone production), and severe degenerative arthritis, all of which contributed to his diminished sense of well-being.

Despite Gregg's ignorance regarding his role in the development of gallstones, he was still responsible for the consequences, including hospitalization and surgery. His thought processes and decisions had led to a damaging lifestyle characterized by poor nutrition and physical activity patterns. These ultimately compromised his gallbladder and liver function, leading to the formation of gallstones. Accepting his mother's statements without questioning them was a passive choice that allowed him to avoid acknowledging the causal role of his actions and remain ignorant of the facts.

According to the Universal Law of Thinking, the quality of our habitual thoughts determines the outcomes and destiny of our lives. In a spiritual sense, thoughts are recognized as the cause and creator of effects. There is a spiritual truth at work beyond what our eyes can perceive, and our thoughts govern our interaction with the spiritual realm. When we understand and consciously align our thoughts with this truth, even in the face of conflicting emotions, we activate its spiritual power. We can transform our mortal situations by aligning our thoughts about our circumstances with a higher reality.

Every thought carries energy and creates something. From a neurological perspective, new thoughts generate new connections within the brain, forming complex neural pathways. On a physical level, thoughts travel at the speed of light, carried by electrons. The energy of thought can be understood through the equation $E=mc^2$. Although the mass of an electron is minuscule, the cumulative effect of repeated thoughts produces significant mass and gives rise to the existence of a new substance. This principle, $E=mc^2$, also forms the foundation of our quantum reality. Through conscious observation and focused attention on a desired outcome, known as the "observer effect," the wave energy function collapses, and the intended manifestation takes material form. We will delve further into this concept when discussing the law of supply.

Moreover, if we perceive excellent health as a tangible entity, it becomes essential to recognize its energetic nature. All substances, including our bodies, are composed of energy and possess a vibrational frequency that can be measured.

Excellent health is associated with a high vibrational energy, while poor health corresponds to a lower frequency. Therefore, the thoughts we cultivate to attain higher levels of health inherently possess better quality. We will delve deeper into this concept in the chapter on the infinite law of increase in health.

Understanding that thinking and thoughts are the primary drivers of our health is of utmost importance. Our thoughts shape our beliefs, actions, and habits, influencing our health and lifestyle. These beliefs, actions, and habits can either be beneficial and empowering, supporting our well-being, or detrimental, leading to irreversible consequences (such as smoking and other self-destructive behaviors that accumulate over time).

When we carefully read these lines, we are infused with the subtle power embedded within the words. The notion conveyed is that from the moment we are born, we possess extraordinary biological abilities that can create any level of health we desire, regardless of our starting point. In my clinical practice, I witness this phenomenon daily among my "biased" patient population, which I define as those who seem more creative and more successful in improving their health because of the empowering support of my team and me. This innate creativity exists within everyone and responds intimately to these universal laws. It often emerges with great vigor in patients facing near-catastrophic clinical situations, both physical and emotional.

We are the creators of our lives, both the art and the

artists!

There are countless ways to express this artistry. However, when it comes to creating our successful health image, it all begins with the initial constructive thought of improvement. The impact of our creative abilities and thoughts on our health is continually confirmed and documented through medical science and technology. For instance, a simple Google Scholar search for the term "stress and disease" yields 3,400,000 scholarly articles. Cancer, heart disease, stroke, diabetes, and hypertension—thousands of clinical trials are exploring the various connections between these conditions and the stressful thoughts we harbor.

Thinking and Its Derivatives

> There is a marvelous inner world that exists within man, and the revelation of such a world enables a man to do, to attain, and to achieve anything he desires within the bounds or limits of Nature. —*Raymond Holliwell, author of Working with the Law: 11 Truth Principles for Successful Living*

So, what are thoughts and ideas? How do we define thinking?

According to Dictionary.com, thought is *"[A]ny conception existing in the mind as the result of mental understanding, awareness, or activity"* or *"any mental representational image of some object or action."*

On the other hand, ideas can be abstract concepts that manifest as mental images, even if our senses do not currently perceive those things. Interestingly, the premise attributed to William James (and Albert Schweitzer) that emerged around five thousand years after a similar conclusion drawn by Hermes Trismegistus (3000-5000 BC) is nearly identical: *"The greatest revolution of our generation is the discovery that human beings, by changing the inner attitudes of their minds, can change the outer aspects of their lives."*

Thinking, then, is the process of generating thoughts. These thoughts are ideas or collections of ideas that are the product of thinking. Although this may sound redundant, it is quite insightful.

Thinking produces various immediate and long-term results:

1) Actions: This is the most direct and immediate outcome of thought. We do not move our hands or feet without a preceding thought, no matter how fleeting or unconscious it may be.

2) Emotions: More complex in nature and appearance, emotions involve the instinctual state of mind. Our experiences and the associated feelings define our thoughtful response. This response is then communicated to other brain areas through holographic patterning, creating three-dimensional images within the brain. Activating the specific regions in this hologram, which may occur repeatedly in certain instances, is based on our past thoughts and current beliefs. These thoughts and beliefs can be positive (promoting health) or negative (detrimental to health).

3) Beliefs: Beliefs are personal truths that arise from our experiences after taking action based on repeated thoughts and actions. Whether the repetitive response affirms or contradicts our initial beliefs determines the formation of these "truths."

Belief is a state of mind in which a person considers something true, whether or not there is empirical evidence to prove its factual certainty. Beliefs can be accepted or held as opinions and involve placing trust or confidence in someone or something. It's important to note that beliefs can be beneficial or detrimental, but they don't necessarily represent the ultimate truth. Beliefs shape our thoughts and conscious activities, leading to actions that produce observable effects, thereby reinforcing or compromising their existence. They are the driving force that motivates our minds to accomplish goals or visualize desired outcomes. Beliefs also influence emotional responses that can impact our health, as we will explore later. Importantly, any desire to change our health or the outcome of an intervention must be accompanied by a reasonable belief, supported by sound thought processes that engage, reinforce, and empower the desired change. For example, if we want to become thinner and fitter, we must tell ourselves and genuinely believe that it is possible, that we know what steps to take, and that we are capable and willing to take those steps. It is unrealistic to expect to achieve these outcomes while constantly telling ourselves or others that we can't be thin or complaining about the difficulty of adopting a fitness mindset.

At Infinite Health Integrative Medicine Center, we orient and empower individuals to focus on their desired health outcomes, believing they are attainable. We assist our patient partners in creating an image that surpasses their initial beliefs and limitations. This empowering approach is based on the actual optimum outcomes that individuals may be completely unaware of during their initial consultations.

Shifting our thoughts from our current state of health to ones that align with our desired outcome requires changing our behavior and energetic focus. Although past experiences may influence our initial goals and beliefs and may feel limited, we must recognize that our bodies are capable of far more than we initially believe. Our vision and sense of empowerment multiply as we experience success and progress toward our goals.

When asked about their limiting beliefs, many individuals new to this mindset express doubt in their ability to achieve their desired goals. Unless these beliefs are changed, they can become self-fulfilling prophecies. However, how can we truly know what we are capable of without challenging ourselves? In many situations, some of us dismiss the possibilities for improvement without giving them a fair chance. I have lost count of the patients who initially said, "I can't," only to achieve positive outcomes, often within a few months.

Henry Ford, a renowned mechanic, once said, *"Whether you believe you can or can't, you're right."* Numerous methods exist to overcome the obstacles that prevent us from achieving optimal health.

An illustrative example is John, a long-term smoker with over sixty pack-years of smoking history. Despite having mild to moderate chronic obstructive pulmonary disease (COPD) and other chronic health issues, John expressed a high motivation level of eight out of ten to improve his health. However, when told that he would need to quit smoking to achieve his desired optimized health, he responded with, *"I can't do that, Doc."*

I thought he would leave the office angry with the staff and me, but we reached an agreement after his lung test results came back. He realized that his limited lung function was severely restricting his activity levels. I reminded him of the impact on EVE (his electronic virtual exercise partner) and what she would continue to do. Remarkably, he quit smoking within four months without any medication. This is a perfect example of how changing a belief that would otherwise compromise an optimized outcome can lead to transformative results.

Continuing our list, thinking also produces:

4) Attitudes: Attitudes result from past thoughts and experiences interacting with similar situations in the present, shaping our favorable or unfavorable disposition toward a person, place, or thing at that moment. It reflects our judgmental ego and is reflected in our behavior. Often, it depends on our perceived benefit at the end of the encounter, whether consciously or subconsciously.

5) Habits: Repeated actions, beliefs, and attitudes become habits, for better or worse. The combination of our multiple habits, attitudes, and beliefs defines our character.

6) Character: Character encompasses the summation of our multiple habits, attitudes, and beliefs.

7) Destiny: By applying our character, which consists of our habits, attitudes, and beliefs, to the events and challenges throughout our lifetime, we determine the outcome, consequences, or destiny of our lives.

The sequence of events described above also applies to our health and well-being. By applying positive thoughts to the challenges that affect our well-being, we can reorient and redefine our health destiny. This demonstrates our ability to determine our health outcomes through the quantum nature of existence. We have constant control over this effect. In the quantum/biocentric reality in which we live, we are both the artists and the art of our lives. We are not mere victims of circumstances, passively observing reality. We are active agents that shape our thoughts, beliefs, and character, influencing ourselves and our environment (our bodies), which are molded by our intentions.

Thoughts, therefore, hold significant power. One hundred years ago, advancements in the basic sciences, led by brilliant physicists like Max Planck, Albert Einstein, Niels Bohr, Werner Heisenberg, and Erwin Schrödinger, revealed that thought and belief directly impact the outcomes of scientific experiments (quantum physics).

"Mind no longer appears to be an accidental intruder into the realm of matter; we ought to rather hail it as the creator and governor of the realm of matter."
  - R.C. Henry, The Mental Universe, Nature 436:29, 2005

Ongoing research on the effects of the mind on health will likely uncover the placebo effect as the quantum/biocentric effect of our minds (thoughts, attitudes, and beliefs) on our well-being. This means that what we think about our health manifests in reality. The biological changes resulting from new constructive thought processes about our health will contribute to healthier outcomes.

Furthermore, the thoughts and beliefs of our "Medical Mastermind" can significantly influence our ability to achieve our desired outcome. The members of our Medical Mastermind may include our physicians, other healthcare providers, and individuals with whom we collaborate harmoniously. The Mastermind provides us with relevant health information and care designed to help us achieve our desired Successful Health Image (SHI).

Our thoughts possess a material creative power, generating new connections between nerves (synapses), new nerve cells (neurons), and new epigenetic modifications of our genes (factors controlling how our DNA expresses itself in more constructive ways). Ultimately, these changes in our bodies mirror the thoughtful modifications we make. They represent personal and behavioral transformations that improve our physical well-being and significantly enhance our health and quality of life.

> *"Imagination is everything. It is the preview of life's coming attractions."*
> *- Albert Einstein*

We are the product of our thoughts, actions, and beliefs up to this moment. Every action we take for our health originates from a preceding thought. Repetitive thoughts about our health, based on similar information, lead to beliefs about our health, which can be beneficial or detrimental depending on the source and reliability of the information. Repetitive actions of a similar nature give rise to health-related habits, which are also influenced by the information and its source. Habits and beliefs shape a specific mental disposition (character) towards excellent or poor health. This disposition determines our fitness destiny across all life situations.

This is why Professor Einstein's quote is so significant. Our imagined ideal of ultimate health and well-being serves as a preview of what we can achieve. Therefore, we must use our Successful Health Image to our greatest advantage.

One of our most important challenges is replacing our knowledge and understanding of our health and establishing new images and thought patterns. Our conscious and subconscious images create the current health reality we hold regarding our well-being, along with the supporting thoughts that contributed to their formation. Even if we are unaware of negative subconscious images undermining our health, we can replace them with positive ones by consciously embedding affirmative patterns in our thoughts and beliefs. Additionally, focusing on our Successful Health Image (SHI) allows us to utilize the Universal Laws of Allowance and Forgiveness, which we will explore later.

Our thoughts and beliefs play a crucial role in our health and our ability to improve it. The healthcare providers who form our Medical Mastermind strongly influence these thoughts and beliefs. The medical parameters related to our ongoing health issues, such as diagnosis, prognosis, and treatment options, are also significantly influenced by the information we receive and how our healthcare providers communicate it. This highlights the critical importance of our Medical Mastermind, as it can either reinforce and empower our thoughts and SHI or weaken and disempower them. We must recognize our responsibility in choosing mentors and advisors who align with our goals and actively support us in achieving our Successful Health Image. Ultimately, it is our responsibility to shape the outcome of our health journey.

Suppose our physician holds a nihilistic attitude characterized by a lack of concern or compassion for our condition and a belief that life has little or no meaning. In that case, seeking another healthcare provider who can work with us in a supportive, harmonious way toward our desired health image is advisable. Some physicians may adopt such an attitude due to their inability to keep up with the vast amount of information in different domains or their unwillingness to explore alternative approaches. Furthermore, we currently face the challenge of interpreting data without fully accounting for quantum or biocentric effects (commonly known as the "placebo/nocebo effect"). This effect, which we will discuss further in chapter four, the Infinite Law of Supply in Health, refers to the influence of an observer's focus and beliefs on the outcome of an observed event. Participants' and investigators' beliefs and attitudes can influence the outcomes of clinical trials. However, addressing this complex issue is still a work in progress.

Lastly, the reactive healthcare paradigm that has emerged in recent decades has led to a system in which patient-practitioner interaction is minimized, resembling an assembly-line process. This shift is partly driven by significantly reduced physician compensation compared with the expo-nential growth in compensation in the pharmaceutical and administrative sectors (e.g., insurance, hospitals).

The academic research literature extensively discusses prac-titioner nihilism in various medical fields, such as neurolog-ical diseases, cancer, vascular and heart diseases, and more. Therefore, when we envision improved health, the advising practitioner must be aware of or willing to review the relevant data. They should also be able to motivate us with patience and compassion, empowering our image to achieve the best possible outcome.

The Successful Health Image (SHI) we create is dynamic and constantly evolving in line with our intentions. We often start our journey with an image reflecting our initial beliefs about what we can achieve. Unfortunately, many of us have encountered reactive physicians whose practice revolves around the insurance model of data interpretation, not fully considering beliefs about the potential for improved outcomes. Breaking free from this paradigm can be challenging for patients. Our culture has long propagated the false promise that we can take a pill without assuming personal responsibility and return to well-being. Many individuals find it difficult to grasp that they are the ultimate creators of their health and reality, and they may not desire to take on that responsibility. However, when we embrace this mindset and reclaim our creative power, we usually have a significant reserve of untapped potential.

When collaborating with an empowering integrative practitioner to shape our ideal health image, we must be open to adapting and refining it as we experience greater success. We must understand that we are responsible for creating our own Medical Mastermind, a team of healthcare professionals who support and enhance our abilities to achieve our health goals. Just as artists refine their outlines and experiment with colors before achieving a final, acceptable image, we should prepare to improve our health image as we progress.

We retrain our thoughts and perspectives by following the guidelines of an empowered, success-oriented program grounded in universal laws. We become more aware of and recognize spontaneous behaviors that do not serve our optimal health while actively seeking out beneficial behaviors that contribute to the well-being of our mind, body, and soul. Most behavioral modification programs require 21 to 261 days to establish new habits, with most individuals falling within the 180 to 250-day range and needing significant support to make the change.

Although research actively dissects the events and biological nature of thinking at macroscopic, microscopic, and molecular biologic levels, we are still in the early stages of understanding these elements. The development of pharmacological interventions and extensive clinical trials will be necessary before we accumulate the robust data required to create truly effective therapeutic interventions for practical settings. Moreover, with technologies such as functional MRI and other imaging methods, we gain clearer insights into the brain regions activated during different emotions and responses to stressors. Therefore, why should we relinquish the power of our bodies and minds to the corporate agendas of the pharmaceutical industry when we have access to such advanced technology?

In addition, studies focus on the molecular and epigenetic changes, such as DNA expression and activity modifiers, that occur during different types of thoughts. While these findings are intriguing, they are still far from yielding a suitable pharmaceutical product that can effectively facilitate sustainable behavioral modification. Realistically, such a "pill" may not replace our innate ability to modify our health-related behavior, especially when a simple, practical, and effective system is available. The potential side effects and toxicities of such a product would require lengthy television advertisements.

Furthermore, pharmaceutical agents are unlikely to have the power to modify our beliefs. This crucial aspect remains within the domain of subconscious suggestion and repetition. When successful, these methods can replace negative behaviors with new constructive ones.

When we reflect on the quote by James Allen and the earlier quote, we understand that our thoughts can prevent illness and help us avoid or heal it by harnessing the power of our minds. By replacing ignorance with knowledge and then applying that knowledge effectively, we actively shape our reality and destiny. This interpretation aligns with the concept of "quantum" and/or "biocentrism" effects in relation to Mr. Allen's thoughts.

Our brains and minds are remarkable tools that serve us and evolve throughout our lives. We can teach and shape them as long as we live. This means we can become the person we choose to be, with the abilities we desire. The key to unlocking this potential lies in identifying and eliminating our limiting thoughts and beliefs. These thoughts and beliefs are either erroneous or based on damaging information. We must replace them with affirmative, empowering ideas that form the foundation of optimal health.

Integrating events and information about our health into our minds significantly shapes our sense of empowerment to achieve wellness. This process unfolds progressively throughout our lives, primarily shaped by the information we receive as children and its quality. It is further reinforced through trial and error as we navigate through life.

Ideally, we would have been best served if we had been exposed to a consistent flow of well-formulated, healthy thoughts grounded in robust, critically peer-reviewed health information from an early age. This information would be continuously updated as we make new health-related decisions that affect our immediate or long-term well-being. However, not all of us had well-informed, objective, caring, and enlightened physicians as parents who could provide us with reliable, up-to-date health information during our childhood. Even if we did, they might not have been available frequently, and the information would likely be outdated by now.

The main point is that action is not initiated until a related idea or thought is formed. These ideas and thoughts are heavily influenced by our beliefs about health and wellness, shaped by our past experiences. The Law of Thinking is conditioned by our beliefs, which influence our thoughts, ideas, decisions, and actions regarding our health.

In our modern lives, most of our thinking is a complex mixture of spontaneous inner dialogue, which I often call chatter or the monkey brain. The constant stream of thoughts constructs our perceived reality, intertwined with egocentric creativity. In many cases, this chatter consists of hypothetical exaggerations. This ego-driven activity is a fertile ground for accumulating misguided thoughts and beliefs that can derail constructive thinking and lead us toward unhealthy behaviors.

Mark Twain once stated that he had experienced many worries, most of which never happened. This highlights that most of our stress and anxiety arises from our imaginations. It's as if the monkey brain is determined to play out endless scenarios of emotionally charged soap operas and violence-filled reality shows for our own (or its own) amusement. Unfortunately, we become the stars of these soap opera fantasies, and our human brains respond to imagined scenarios like they would to real-life situations. This means that our bodies undergo the same physiological stress response whether a literal saber-toothed tiger stands before us or exists only in the "screen" of our mind.

So, what happens to our bodies when we respond to stress? As we think—since we are almost always thinking about something due to the constant chatter—our brains provide us (or our minds) with a synthesis of information based on the integration of sensory perceptions. Our minds, influenced by past experiences, filter and integrate this information. However, the mind is also quite creative and can create or imagine situations that feel just as real as actual experiences. Therefore, our minds are not particularly critical or discerning when distinguishing between sensory input and imagination-generated input.

Any disruption in the equilibrium between an organism and its environment is called "stress." Stressors can arise from information received by the brain's cortex through sensory organs, or our imaginations can create them. These stressors are assessed as either threatening or non-threatening and are forwarded to the amygdala, the brain's emotional center. The emotional message is then relayed to the hypothalamus, which activates the autonomic and parasympathetic nervous systems. These nervous pathways send signals to various body organs, such as increasing heart rate or changing blood pressure, to elicit bodily responses. The hypothalamus also releases multiple hormones that further communicate with the pituitary gland, initiating a cascade of hormonal messages throughout the body. These responses perpetuate the brain's interpretation of stress.

Depending on the duration of the stress, whether acute or chronic, the hypothalamus releases different hormones. These hormones include corticotropin-releasing hormone (CRH), antidiuretic hormone (ADH), gonadotropin-releasing hormone (GnRH), and thyrotropin-releasing hormone (TRH). These hormones, in turn, stimulate the release of adrenocorticotropic hormone (ACTH), growth hormone (GH), thyroid-stimulating hormone (TSH), prolactin, 8-lipotropin, 3-endorphin, follicle-stimulating hormone (FSH), and luteinizing hormone (LH) from their respective glands. This hormonal cascade creates an optimal bodily environment to sustain survival in the face of a perceived threat, similar to when a saber-toothed tiger attacks.

During acute stress reactions, one of the main hormones released by the adrenal glands in response to ACTH is cortisol. Cortisol regulates blood pressure and glucose levels, keeping the body alert and vigilant. It inhibits insulin activity, resulting in higher blood sugar levels that can be immediately utilized as an energy source. Chronic stress and the prolonged release of cortisol due to ongoing adrenal stimulation are associated with the exacerbation of diabetes, hypertension, and severe immune compromise, which may accelerate cancer progression.

The next significant hormones released during a stress response are the catecholamine derivatives, mainly epinephrine (adrenaline) and norepinephrine. These hormones have various effects on the body. They increase blood flow to the heart, brain, and skeletal muscles and widen the airways to improve breathing. Additionally, they promote sodium retention by the kidneys, leading to increased blood volume and improved blood flow to vital organs. During the fight-or-flight response, catecholamines tend to reduce blood flow to organs that are less essential in that moment (after all, worrying about our kidneys or skin appearance is not a priority when facing a grizzly bear).

Moreover, both epinephrine and norepinephrine inhibit the action of insulin and increase the availability of sugar as an energy source (sweet-and-sour sauce for the tiger?). Adversarial stress responses also result in decreased levels of thyroid hormones, insulin, and the gonadotropins follicle-stimulating hormone (FSH) and luteinizing hormone (LH), while growth hormone and prolactin levels are increased. It is worth noting that chronic stress can disrupt the menstrual cycle and impair reproductive function in women.

Similarly, men may experience significant reductions in testosterone levels due to decreased FSH and LH under similar circumstances (who needs libido when dodging claws?). While acute stress causes a significant increase in growth hormone levels, chronic stress leads to decreased growth hormone production and secretion. This is particularly important for the body's ability to repair itself.

In 2007, Cohen, Janicki-Deverts, and Miller published an article in the Journal of the American Medical Association (JAMA) discussing the effects of psychological stress on disease. They highlighted that chronic stress can have detrimental effects on various hormones, leading to the worsening of chronic diseases such as chronic fatigue, hypertension, obesity, diabetes, anxiety, irritability, and depression. It can also affect metabolic and reproductive functions, including infertility, and compromise the immune system.

Regarding clinical outcomes, our focus is more on the potential adverse effects of our illness. This is often the result of our own misconceptions or limited interactions with healthcare providers. We tend to dwell on the adverse side effects of medications or anything that may worsen our well-being, and these thoughts linger in our minds.

Consequently, our confidence is undermined, and our trust is eroded. Anxiety and fear of unfavorable outcomes occupy our attention. However, when we can shift our focus towards positive and constructive outcomes, we can reduce the repetitive activation of the stress response. This, in turn, enhances the body's natural healing tendencies and encourages the immune system to work in harmony with ongoing therapies.

To foster a proactive and positive mindset, different approaches are necessary. Relying solely on medications is unlikely to achieve this mindset. Medications can dull our perceptions and hinder our ability to assess challenges coherently. As an oncologist, I have observed this phenomenon among my patients over the years. Some struggle to shift their mindset and thought patterns towards a more constructive and positive outlook. Consequently, they may experience unfavorable outcomes despite receiving effective pharmaceutical support. Adverse prognoses from misinformed family members or nihilistic and uninformed physicians can significantly impact survival and quality of life, even when patients respond well to treatment.

James Allen, the author of "Out from the Heart," emphasizes the power of the mind to shape one's life. Understanding that our thoughts and mindset are malleable and can be modified through patient effort empowers us to gain complete control over our thoughts and ultimately achieve liberation.

In this context, we should consider the benefits of the Law of Thinking. This universal principle recognizes thought as an unchanging, repetitive process that determines the life conditions and destinies of both men and women. Consequently, the quality of our dominant thoughts and their consequences directly impact our health.

If you have been motivated to read "Think and Live Longer" for a specific reason, it is precisely that reason that will enable you to achieve the desired success in your health journey. Do you believe there is a better version of yourself within you, longing for a higher quality of life, improved energy levels, better physical fitness, a happier sex life, and the ability to be more active and vibrant? We recognize our unique capacity for change, supported by concepts such as the Law of Supply, the multiple worlds interpretation of quantum mechanics, quantum entanglement, and biocentricism. By activating this belief, we set in motion the means to attain our desired outcomes in motion. It is not only about changing our thoughts regarding our health and controlling them to facilitate the desired transformation—freeing ourselves from the monkey brain, catastrophic thinking, and constant chatter.

To empower ourselves on the path to optimal health, we need a practical framework or guidelines to achieve positive outcomes and avoid negative ones. This is where "Think and Live Longer" comes into play.

James Allen eloquently states that the nature of the mind is to create its conditions and choose the states in which it resides. Moreover, the mind can alter any condition and discard any state, continuously making choices and gaining exhaustive experiences from different states.

Your vision represents the future version of yourself that you aspire to become, while your ideal serves as a prophecy of your ultimate potential. In Luke 17:21, Jesus speaks of the kingdom of God residing within us, which can be understood as the nature of our inner consciousness and the thoughts we consistently maintain, whether consciously or subconsciously. It is interconnected with our state of mindfulness. The more peaceful, constructive, healthy, and organized our consciousness, the more we will experience a perfected and conscious life akin to a heavenly existence.

These empowered thoughts are the same ones that lead us to optimal health. By guiding our thoughts with mindfulness, enlightenment, and productivity, we pave the way for achieving all our aspirations. This guidance aligns with the message in Matthew 6:33, where we are encouraged to seek the Kingdom of Heaven, a conscious state of mindfulness, and trust that all things will be added to us. This insightful guidance emphasizes that attaining a heavenly state of consciousness requires an orderly, disciplined mind focused on the desirable qualities of empowered, enlightened thinking rather than fixating on the mundane needs of daily life. The extrapolation for our health journey is the same. Our mindful, enlightened, and informed thoughts and ideas lead us to our desired well-being destination.

The mandate is clear: we must align our thinking with and focus on using universal laws to achieve excellent health outcomes. Being attuned to these qualities empowers and guides us toward the gifts of the universe—perfect healing and fitness. If we can maintain an organized, disciplined, and proactive vision of our positive and happy endgame, excellence in health, we will more easily achieve it. This echoes the wisdom in the James Allen quote mentioned earlier.

However, if we allow ourselves to be easily distracted, driven by emotions, short-tempered, prideful, envious, or engage in unconscious, self-serving, and unenlightened thoughts and behaviors, we will experience unpleasant outcomes. These results will be out of harmony with universal laws and not aligned with our ultimate well-being. From a quantum interpretation perspective, such thoughts would impose adversity on an individual's thought system. Losing sight of our health vision due to distractions, whether emotional or otherwise, is akin to an athlete losing focus on their dominant performance and, consequently, losing a race or tournament. This failure to "keep an eye on the prize" typically leads to temporary setbacks or failure. The key to achieving excellent health, especially during recovery from illness, lies in cultivating a positive self-image through organized, affirmative thinking. Proverbs 23:7 states, *"As a man thinketh in his heart, so is he,"* and Job noted in Job 3:25, *"What I feared has come upon me; what I dreaded has happened to me."* These verses highlight the adverse outcomes resulting from fixating on fear or dread.

James Allen's words remind us that our vision and ideals hold the promise of our future selves. By nurturing a mindful and empowered consciousness, guided by universal laws and enlightened thinking, we unlock the potential for excellent health and realize our true selves.

These quotes highlight the impact of thoughts on our existence and our role as biocentrists or quantum participants in shaping the determinism of our lives. They also imply the power of the mental principle of transmutation, which refers to the ability to change from one form to another. This transmutation occurs when we persistently think about desired or undesired outcomes until they eventually manifest in our lives.

While this principle may seem straightforward, it is poorly understood, particularly when considering the prevalent chronic disease processes contributing to a significant portion of healthcare expenditures, surpassing $2.5 trillion annually and continuing to rise. Our current health paradigm appears to endorse a path that leads to debilitating chronic healthcare problems. The United States spends over 16% of its gross domestic product on healthcare, making it the world's largest spender. The next-closest competitor allocates only six percent. These statistics reveal the substantial financial investment in healthcare, despite the country's relatively low overall health outcomes compared to other nations.

During a discussion with a new patient about his pain and healing issues, the significance of thinking and thoughts became strikingly evident to me. This patient was dealing with moderate to severe degenerative arthritis, peripheral vascular disease, and peripheral neuropathy (nerve damage). The underlying causes of his peripheral neuropathy and vascular disease were linked to long-standing diabetes, which, in turn, stemmed from chronic morbid obesity and an indulgent lifestyle. Degenerative arthritis could be traced back to osteoporosis resulting from vitamin D deficiency, hypogonadism, and a history of tobacco abuse. When reflecting on the causality of his pain, the patient adamantly declared, *"It's not my fault!"*

While I don't always approach patients in such an aggressive manner, using these laws requires an understanding of how our thoughts, shaped by accurate and comprehensive knowledge, influence our health outcomes. Therefore, I engaged in a discussion with this young man about his eating habits, two-pack-per-day smoking habit, diabetes, and hypercholesterolemia, outlining how his thinking, even if misinformed, and subsequent nutritional and lifestyle choices had contributed to poor health.

Through compassionate discussions and targeted practices

such as imaging exercises, a meditation on health, and biofeedback training, our team provided education that sufficiently altered his thinking paradigm. As a result, he successfully created a new image of health for himself.

* * *

The Think and Live Longer Mind Shift Hack: Establishing a Daily Meditation Practice

Meditating daily has been scientifically proven to offer numerous health benefits, including:

- Lowering high blood pressure.
- Reducing blood lactate levels can alleviate anxiety and anxiety attacks.
- Decreasing tension-related pain, such as tension headaches, insomnia, and joint issues.
- Increasing serotonin production can improve mood and behavior.
- Strengthening the immune system.
- Boosting energy levels.
- Inducing alpha brainwave patterns that promote self-healing.
- Enhancing emotional stability.
- Increasing levels of happiness.
- Cultivating clarity and peace of mind.
- Sharpening cognitive abilities.
- Alleviating feelings of instability and being overwhelmed.

To start experiencing these tremendous health benefits, follow these steps:

Aim to meditate twice daily for a minimum of 15 minutes per session. However, if your schedule doesn't allow for that, meditating once a day will still yield benefits.

The optimal times for meditation are either in the morning before starting your day or before bedtime. Cultivating this habit is key.

One common challenge when beginning meditation is dealing with a wandering mind. It's completely normal and should not discourage you. The mind requires training. If your thoughts are drifting, redirect your attention to your breathing or the self-healing imagery (SHI) you created from the previous chapter. You'll notice your mind wandering less with practice; those 15 minutes will pass quickly.

As additional support, consider listening to binaural beats while meditating. These beats facilitate your mind's transition into the theta state. You can find free binaural beat audio/videos on platforms like YouTube and the products available at EOC Institute.

Another effective approach for beginners is to use guided meditations. These provide a focus by following the imagery presented by the guide. Below is a partial script from previous group meditation classes at Infinite Health Integrative Medicine Center. It may be helpful to record yourself reading this meditation and play it back during your meditation sessions.

THE INFINITE HEALTH-GUIDED MEDITATION

Begin by relaxing in a quiet, soothing environment. You may sit in a chair or lie on your bed; get into a comfortable position where you will not be disturbed.

Close your eyes.
Inhale a deep breath to the count of four.
Hold that breath to the count of four.
Release the breath to the count of six.
Again, inhale a deep breath to the count of four.
Hold that breath to the count of four.
Release the breath to the count of six.
One more time, inhale a deep breath to the count of four.
Hold that breath to the count of four.
Release the breath to the count of six.
Now, imagine you have magically been transported to your favorite location - the place that offers you the most peace, the most relaxation.
This may be an island beach, a cabin in the snow-covered mountains, or even the rocking chair on your front porch, enjoying the sunrise.
Wherever brings you the most peace is perfect for you.
This is your private space.
Your time here is your own.
You are free from all responsibilities at this moment.

All is well.
It is safe and good for you to be in this space right now.
Fully engage all of your senses.
Notice the colors of the scenery.
How bright and beautiful is the sun or the moon?
What brilliant colors are shimmering in the ocean?
Or, how lush and green is the grass, and what colors are the flowers in the field?
Tune in to the sounds.
Do you hear birds singing?
Do you hear waves rolling and out again?
Do you hear the wind whipping in the air?
Notice how you feel.
Is the sun warming your face?
Is the wind gently teasing your hair?
How does the ground feel beneath your feet?
Notice the aromas.
Do you smell honeysuckle?
Do you smell salty air?
Do you smell pine trees?
Or, do you smell coffee beans roasting?
Spend a few minutes here, breathing slowly and deeply in this place of sweet serenity;
This place of security;
This beautiful place where all is well.

.

.

.

When you are ready, notice someone in the distance walking towards you.
There is a familiarity about them.

But you are not quite sure who it is.

As this person walks towards you, getting closer and closer, you can see her/his smiling face.

She/he seems genuinely happy and at peace with everything.

When his person is standing in front of you, you realize she/he is you.

You, in your MOST vibrant, MOST energetic, and MOST healthy physical state of being.

Notice how the ideal version of you appears.

Notice how your body is toned, fit, and youthful-looking.

Notice your clear, glowing skin.

Your hair is shiny, healthy, and strong.

See yourself smiling radiantly, joyfully.

You are at peace with yourself.

You are at peace with the world.

.

.

.

Now, imagine merging with this ideal, infinite version of yourself.

You are now one.

Notice how you feel in your ideal state of optimized health.

Notice how much more energy you have.

Notice how easy it is to move, to walk, to run, and even to jump.

Notice how full of peace and joy you are.

Notice how wonderful, happy, and in love you are with yourself, your body, and your life.

You are now in your optimized state of physical, emotional, mental, and spiritual health,

Right here, right now.

Breathe this in deeply.

Stay in this space for a few minutes, really breathing deeply.

Feel and know that this is who you already are.

.

.

.

When you are ready, bring your awareness back into your physical body.

Wiggle your fingers and toes.

Open your eyes.

Elongate your back.

Take a deep breath in and release.

Reach your hands up to the sky and get a good stretch.

Congratulations! You are now one step closer to retraining your mind to think in ways that support your goals for optimal health and longevity.

The Infinite Law of Empowered Perspective and Health: The Notion of the "Medical Mastermind" and the Case for Mindfulness

"A Mastermind may be created through the bringing together or blending,
in a spirit of perfect harmony, of two or more minds.
Out of this harmonious blending, the chemistry of the
mind creates a third mind which may be appropriated
and used by one or all of the individual minds."
-Napoleon Hill, The Law of Success, 1928

What are the key elements that empower us to pursue improved outcomes? Which elements are helpful, and which ones offer little or negative benefits?

Given the abundance of scientific information, mentors and knowledgeable clinicians are essential for those who wish to avoid the consequences of not understanding what constitutes optimal health. Access to these experts will lead us to form thoughts and beliefs that significantly improve well-being and therapeutic outcomes. As the artists of our lives, we must remain vigilant in welcoming thoughts, actions, habits, and character traits that bring benefits.

Motivational and mindfulness techniques are currently being studied as complementary approaches to optimized medical management for various diseases. While this represents progress, it also presents challenges. This is because the quality of life and other experiences resulting from these techniques are subjective and harder to measure than physiological or survival endpoints.

For instance, positive outcomes from these techniques may be attributed to the simple effect of "caring," which, in my observation, is, unfortunately, lacking in most patient-physician interactions nowadays. While I would like to blame the evolution of medical economics and healthcare delivery for this problem, ultimately, it remains the responsibility of healthcare providers to provide genuine care.

Under the current medical delivery paradigm, physicians are often rewarded more for their technical expertise and efficiency in prescribing medications or performing procedures than for their compassion. However, I have found that a physician's ability to convey care, understanding, acceptance, humor, and happiness positively impacts patients. William James, who studied to be a physician in the 1860s, expressed a similar view on the use of pharmaceuticals. He believed that a doctor's presence and moral influence on the patient and their family were often more significant than anything else, except surgery.

Although pharmaceuticals have advanced significantly since James' time, we still face similar uncertainties. Until we can precisely tailor pharmaceutical treatments to specific clinical entities based on defined genomic factors, it is the thought of healing and health that physicians impress upon our minds, giving hope and belief and invoking the quantum/biocentric effect for every patient. Let's now examine another case that will help us define the origin, goals, and purpose of the Medical Mastermind.

Joan, a fifty-six-year-old mid-level executive, came to me seeking help for multiple medical problems after being evaluated by several other healthcare providers over the past six years. These providers had diagnosed her with various conditions, including Lupus, rheumatoid arthritis, Crohn's disease, ulcerative colitis, fibromyalgia, irritable bowel syndrome, diabetes, degenerative arthritis, hypertension, hypothyroidism, sleep apnea, anxiety, depression, and multiple blood lipid abnormalities. Joan had accepted the notion of a progressively chronic disease negatively impacting her well-being and potentially shortening her lifespan compared to her healthier siblings.

At age thirty-two, Joan underwent a complete hysterectomy and was advised to discontinue hormone therapies due to the perceived risk of cancer and heart disease. She was prescribed numerous pharmaceuticals by different physicians in an attempt to manage her symptoms. After a brief examination and discussion, Joan reached her breaking point when her primary internist prescribed yet another medication to regulate her glucose metabolism.

When Joan came to see me, she was frustrated with the number of prescription medications she was taking and her persistent mild obesity, despite her passion for road biking. After conducting a comprehensive metabolic and hormone laboratory analysis, the results revealed suboptimal hormone and metabolite levels and evidence of liver damage.

Based on these findings, I designed a comprehensive precision treatment program to address Joan's health challenges. After six to eight weeks on the program, her blood sugar levels significantly decreased, and she was able to discontinue her anti-anxiety and antidepressant medications. Joan experienced a notable increase in overall well-being, improved sleep patterns, and the complete resolution of her fibromyalgia and irritable bowel/colitis symptoms.

Furthermore, her liver function tests returned to normal, and her hemoglobin A1C, a measure of average blood sugar levels, dropped from 9.2 to 7.0 (the normal range being 4.8 to 5.6). By the fourth month of follow-up, her liver tests remained normal, and her A1C was no longer in the diabetic range at 5.9, even though she had stopped all diabetes medications six weeks earlier. Joan continued biking with increasing enthusiasm and aimed to complete her first Century ride (100 miles) around five months after her initial visit. Her average speed had increased from twelve to 15.6 miles per hour on her last twenty-mile ride before the century event in 2017.

Four months later, Joan's diabetes, hypertension, depressive symptoms, liver function abnormalities, body aches, and joint pain had all resolved without the need for further medication. At the one-year mark, she continued to improve her fitness and now challenged her husband on speed and endurance, motivating him to become a patient as well. Joan and her husband cycled the twenty-mile circuit at speeds ranging from 19.6 to 19.8 miles per hour.

Given these remarkable improvements, the question arose: How did Joan realize a complete resolution of her diabetes, metabolic syndrome, steatohepatitis, depression, gastrointestinal colitis syndrome, fibromyalgia, and arthritic complaints in just five or six months?

Joan would enthusiastically attribute her successful outcomes to creating a positive health image and the empowering motivational mindfulness exercises that facilitated constructive thoughts, decisions, and focus. She would also acknowledge the valuable role of her physician (yours truly) to some extent.

So, how can we make the most of our health during our time on this physical plane? The answer is straightforward: We establish a Medical Mastermind as our empowered medical mentor and collaborator in making decisions that optimize our well-being. The Medical Mastermind refers to a health-care team formed and brought together by the individual to achieve successful health outcomes.

When Joan first came to see me, it was clear that her medical mastermind was not aligned with the health vision she wanted to create for herself. Although Joan knew what she didn't want - an ongoing decline in health - she hadn't yet formulated her successful health image (SHI). The turning point came during her last doctor's visit when she was offered additional medications to combat her deteriorating health. The combination of uncertainty about her future well-being and fear propelled her to seek decisive change. Defining the SHI proved somewhat challenging, as she recognized the need for advice and guidance to attain her optimal outcome. This marked the intuitive beginning of her search for a Medical Mastermind (MM). Finding knowledgeable, compassionate, sympathetic, and like-minded team members to support her success was the crucial first step toward achieving her goals. This infrastructure is available to all of us as we strive to create our empowered health, and compromising in its acquisition should not be accepted.

The most significant factor in Joan's successful health image was its creation. This is the essence of the Medical Master-mind: it enables an exponential collaborative increase in the knowledge base for all participants. Joan learned from the Medical Mastermind that an empowered, successful health image is a personal, dynamic creation that can be refined at any time. Her previous experiences had constrained her thoughts and beliefs, limiting her ultimate vision of success. She gradually reviewed and transformed many of these limiting convictions throughout her subsequent victories. For example, she initially found it amusing to contemplate an average biking speed of fifteen miles per hour, yet she is now approaching twenty miles per hour. An important challenge for Joan was reconciling her desired health outcomes with their appearance. The appearance of these goals (the image) not only signifies that we can achieve them (and we certainly can) but also indicates that they already exist energetically, waiting for us to call them forth by using the universal laws.

Natural science is not merely a description and explanation of nature; it is an integral part of the interplay between nature and ourselves, as expressed by Werner Heisenberg, Nobel Laureate in Physics.

Belief is the key driver (creative force) in this context, as it motivates, influences, and shapes our vision into the final outcome. It serves as the quantum (or biocentric) assistant in creating the reality of health for all of us, just as it did for Joan. As she began experiencing one success after another in relation to her health image, she progressively empowered her outcomes, replacing her limiting beliefs with increasing motivation, desire, and focused intent.

The vision, image, or thought that we create with the support of our healthcare providers, coaches, or partners (the Medical Mastermind) should serve as our empowered promise to ourselves. The optimized state of health we agree upon, guided by their expertise, becomes the prediction of what we will ultimately achieve. There is no room for compromise, and our minds drive our pursuit of this vision. The outcome we attain results from the quantum-based clinical effect that emerges from the partnership and collective effort of both the patient and the clinicians. This collaborative approach is the essence of integrative care, where action over time and distance, fueled by the energy of thought and belief, leads to tangible clinical effects.

From a transformational perspective, we are nurturing a clinical effect arising from the quantum clinical input of both the patient and the participants in the Medical Mastermind. Through this methodology, we provide ourselves with a means of empowered individual self-development and enlightenment, guided by principles for personal success. Simultaneously, we take ownership of the self-directed pursuit of extraordinary physical, spiritual, and intellectual health. The thoughts that develop from the mastermind, mentorship, exercises, and readings guide the body toward improved longevity.

The quality of thought plays a pivotal role in the manifestation of the Law of Thinking in health. It tells us that our dominant state of mind, encompassing our beliefs, attitudes, and more, shapes our life experiences and, specifically, our health. What we genuinely believe, based on well-informed perspectives, is what we will witness in terms of our health. Put simply, what we consistently think about regarding our health will materialize.

However, we must not assume that a brief thirty-minute or even thirty-hour exploration of a health issue on WebMD or "Dr. Google" is sufficient to fully understand the current thinking and practices on the topic. While information on a particular subject may appear straightforward in online chat rooms where laypeople discuss their treatment outcomes, achieving the best possible results often requires subtle adjustments and optimization of various parameters by a skilled, experienced practitioner. This clinical finesse is often the culmination of a career-long process of trial and error, heavily influenced by the complexity of each individual and their unique healthcare concerns. Hence, the significance of the Medical Mastermind and the harmonious collaboration among its participants in achieving optimal outcomes becomes apparent.

It is logical to exercise caution when interpreting clinical trial findings, given historical instances in which misinterpretation of data and its generalizations have led to adverse outcomes for the wider population. For example, the FDA's previous recommendation of the "food pyramid" underwent significant changes approximately two years ago. This illustrates the perplexing nature of misguided thinking. When a flawed belief structure or failure to heed an experienced advisor's advice results in poor outcomes.

Take, for example, the erroneous conception of the old food pyramid, which advocated avoiding cholesterol and saturated fats. It was not aligned with the greater good as intended for humanity. We have witnessed the consequences of this misinterpretation in the form of an epidemic of obesity and diabetes in both children and adults, accompanied by numerous complications associated with these conditions. Ultimately, this misguided decision led to increased instances of heart disease, vascular problems, and immune disorders, as well as higher rates of cancer and dementia. Therefore, our thoughts are effective only when they align with what is universally recognized as beneficial. It is a process of trial and error that can yield substantial benefits, provided it adheres to the universal good.

Your vision of health should harmonize with and be pursued in accordance with what is universally accepted as good. Are physicians always infallible in this regard? Clearly not. However, a well-informed and optimized health image can be achieved through conscientious collaboration between physicians, their patient partners, and other members of their Medical Mastermind. The involved physicians can provide the balanced guidance and mentorship necessary to minimize deviations and errors in interpreting the available information.

> *When we change our thinking for the better, we automatically change our lives for the better. ... A change of thought must precede every change in the life (health) and in the affairs of man, when our intention becomes reconciled or cooperative with the universal (God's) intentions, then we become an expression of that good. This is working with the law.*
> —Raymond Holliwell, author of Working with the
> Law:
> 11 Truth Principles for Successful Living

One significant challenge we face is understanding the root causes of our health problems. Often, a medical issue or symptom can be attributed to multiple factors, not solely hereditary issues. More commonly, these factors stem from self-imposed stress (as indicated by insurance company data, which shows that only 10-25% of health issues result from genetics, while 75-90% stem from lifestyle choices) or from misguided beliefs, known as limiting thoughts.

To address our health challenges, we need support and a plan that empowers us to make positive changes. This involves utilizing available information resources and engaging with a Medical Mastermind—a team of physicians or well-trained healthcare practitioners experienced in comprehensive integrative care. Through their transformative mentorship and collaborative guidance, they help us identify counter-productive behaviors and the limiting beliefs that underlie them. In essence, these practitioners become our counselors of transformation and successful empowerment. They instill a kind of thinking that ultimately drives positive change, because the origin of our outcomes in this quantum/biocentric reality. Empowered thoughts aligned with optimal well-being become the driving force behind positive change and the attainment of the great health we deserve.

Focusing our attention and contemplation on healthy outcomes directs the constructive quantum energy of belief and intention toward our vision of well-being. This has a constructive, beneficial effect, positively changing our observed environment. Keeping our thoughts organized, disciplined, and constructive is crucial, as misguided information and anecdotes often permeate the medical literature. Awareness of their presence and the abundance of pseudo-medical products in the wellness marketplace helps us make informed choices and is a byproduct of our engagement with the Medical Mastermind.

Additionally, we must remember the mischievous "monkey brain" that constantly seeks to implant contrary and ignorant images in our minds. These images are just as easily produced as the healthy ones. Therefore, following a personalized plan crafted by a skilled integrative medicine practitioner is highly beneficial. Such a practitioner understands how to achieve optimized health by providing necessary accountability. When reviewing and integrating universal laws with their patients, guidance and mentorship play a pivotal role in achieving motivational success and improving health outcomes. This approach fosters compliance and overall self-awareness in receptive patients.

In essence, each of us can control the outcomes of our lives and health through the discipline and content of our thoughts. So, when we choose to consume deep-fried chicken, we should not expect to avoid the risk of stroke or acute coronary syndrome.

Our awareness of well-being and natural alignment with it shape our perspective and provide an overarching view of health, leading to the manifestation of our successful health image. As we focus our thoughts on this vision and its benefits, our conscious self-awareness emits energy that, when combined with subconscious forces, attracts similar energies, vibrations, and thoughts. This sets a series of events and actions in motion that culminate in the desired outcome—excellent health. Remaining open-minded and receptive to the potential benefits of our collaborative interventions often yields even greater benefits than we initially anticipated.

Participating in a structured program incorporating guided imagery and biofeedback can benefit individuals facing health challenges. Guided imagery involves a trained practitioner guiding the patient-partner in creating specific mental images that engage all the senses. On the other hand, biofeedback is a process of increasing awareness and control over physiological functions using instruments that provide information on those functions. The best outcomes are achievable by combining these scientifically proven complementary techniques with patient education and behavior modification coursework in a supportive environment. This program cultivates consistent, disciplined, and empowered thinking, acting as a beacon that emits a homing signal for the desired outcome—or even something better. Even subtle mental efforts contribute to the desired outcome through the power of empowering thoughts and beliefs applied to one's life.

When we discipline ourselves to organize our thinking process around thoughts that align with our ultimate health goals, our minds can effortlessly work toward achieving that vision. This taps into our creativity and changes our bodies' healing physiology. By finalizing the vision and committing to the expected positive change, we unleash the powerful transformational destiny. The quality of our end product is determined by the quality and focus of our beliefs, vision, and effort, regardless of our starting point.

From a practical standpoint, we can address our thoughts on two levels:

Level 1: Old Thinking

This refers to the limiting beliefs deeply ingrained in our subconscious mind that may hinder our progress toward better health. It is crucial to identify and understand these limiting beliefs, which can originate from various sources such as parental and societal influences. These beliefs act as metaphorical balls and chains, undermining our efforts for improvement and sabotaging our present and future well-being. They are the foundation of the critical and wandering thoughts of the "monkey brain." The empowerment process aims to equip patient partners with tools that transform their belief structures into passionate allies to pursue good health. Specifically designed exercises aim to foster empowered self-realization of well-being by increasing awareness of the origins of limiting beliefs and removing the barriers they impose, whether they formed in childhood or later in life.

Level 2: Current Thinking

To understand our current health, we must examine each aspect of our well-being and identify any thoughts that hinder healing and improvement. It is crucial to consistently hold an image of our optimal health outcome, especially if we start from a state of deficiency. This means recognizing and replacing negative thoughts and beliefs that may be causally related to our diagnoses, anticipated outcomes, and treatment plans. Negative thoughts, beliefs, and behaviors can potentially exacerbate medical conditions due to the physiological stress responses they elicit. These limiting thoughts and beliefs play a significant role because they reflect anticipated health outcomes communicated to the field of pure health potentiality, which in turn influences our overall health and well-being.

We contribute to our perception of health reality by focusing on and affirming the accuracy and validity of each diagnosis we receive. Whether it's a simple bone fracture or a complex autoimmune disease like systemic lupus erythematosus, our belief in the possibility of successful resolution shapes the efforts we are willing to make for change. Once we have completed an inventory of our health issues, which may seem never-ending for many of us, it is essential to create a vision of complete resolution and a fresh outcome. Only then can we nurture these images with our sincere efforts and beliefs.

Let's take diabetes as an example. This chronic disease, influenced by multiple factors, stems from inadequate blood glucose control by the hormone insulin. Simply put, we either have insufficient insulin to regulate glucose, or the available quantity cannot perform its role effectively. Regarding the current diabetes epidemic, our bodies have been challenged by the excessive consumption of carbohydrate-rich diets, as advocated by the FDA until their recommendations were updated in 2014 due to the rise of obesity, diabetes, and cardiovascular diseases. Remarkably, the American Diabetes Association still recommends a high-carbohydrate diet. However, I discontinued prescribing these detrimental nutritional regimens years ago. As a result, I have witnessed complete improvements in abnormal hemoglobin A1C levels among compliant patients. By eliminating inappropriate foods from their dietary lifestyles, these patients have saved significant amounts of money on pharmaceutical costs and avoided numerous adverse drug reactions associated with oral hypoglycemic medications and insulin.

When we consume carbohydrates, the rapid increase in blood

glucose triggers the release of endorphins and serotonin, which have calming and mood-enhancing effects. This is often referred to as "comfort food" and is used as a therapeutic measure to alleviate negative emotions such as loneliness, sadness, depression, and guilt caused by stressful situations. However, this type of nutritional intake can be both a form of self-medication and self-sabotage. Some patients may experience difficulties when trying to withdraw from the mood-enhancing effects of neurotransmitters like serotonin, beta-endorphins, dopamine, and norepinephrine. In certain cases, medication typically used for narcotic withdrawal may be necessary to assist with withdrawing from these foods. Understanding this challenging hormonal environment during withdrawal is where mind-body-directed imaging techniques and biofeedback truly find their place.

Considering the Infinite Law of Thinking in relation to health, it is clear that deviating from known beneficial nutritional pathways will only lead to undesired physical attributes and biological outcomes, such as obesity, metabolic syndrome, and diabetes. These conditions further contribute to medical problems and compromise the quality of life and health span. Conversely, by consistently maintaining a focus on the qualities and benefits of a healthy nutritional lifestyle, we can create a consistently beneficial internal environment in our bodies and reap the rewards of these ideas.

Incorporating guided imagery, motivational techniques, and therapeutic interventions into medicine has gradually gained acceptance over the past few decades. Dr. Herbert Benson's pioneering studies played a significant role in promoting these techniques to conventional physicians. More recently, clinical trials incorporating mind-body components such as guided imagery, meditation, and motivational enhancement have objectively demonstrated substantial improvements in outcomes. Guided imagery involves directing one's thoughts or mental images toward relaxation and a desired outcome or state of being. This is often facilitated by auditory programming and, occasionally, by complementary subliminal visual videos. The body, responding to these sensory inputs, perceives them as originating from external sources and reacts accordingly.

Many guided imagery techniques employ auditory enhancements to synchronize brainwave activity, promoting relaxation and subconscious imprinting. Some studies have even shown improved immune system function as a result. Personally, I have observed improved patient engagement and participation when utilizing directed imagery techniques that incorporate binaural auditory brainwave methodologies (brainwave entrainment). Even initially reluctant patients recognize the benefits of these techniques and become more dedicated to the program. Visual subconscious programs also use brainwave modulations to enhance therapeutic interventions. Numerous studies have consistently demonstrated positive outcomes in various areas, notably pain reduction, stress reduction for stress-related disorders, and hypertension. Dr. Benson's initial studies on the effects of meditation focused on hypertension.

Additional positive outcomes have been observed in studies for congestive heart failure, acute coronary syndrome, stroke prevention and rehabilitation, obesity, smoking cessation, and the treatment of other substance addictions such as narcotics and alcohol. Lastly, anxiety, depression, and panic disorders all respond more significantly to a mind-body component. Medical professionals and patients alike are confirming the utility of the infinite Law of Thinking. We can significantly enhance and balance our lives by simply reflecting on what we want and how we want to live, while maintaining a crisp, clear picture at both the conscious and subconscious levels.

The Law of Empowered Perspective primarily centers on the quality of our habitual thoughts and how we approach mindfulness and thoughtful consideration in our decision-making. The crucial aspect lies in assessing this quality, which requires an awareness of our thought processes. By adopting a mindful perspective and being aware of our thoughts, particularly when making life decisions, we position ourselves for more incredible benefits.

This is because we can better evaluate our competency and the extent of our knowledge base, akin to an "executive view." Executives make informed decisions after considering information from competent and knowledgeable support staff and mentors. Simultaneously, as we maintain a mindful perspective on our thoughts and potential actions to achieve excellent health outcomes, our focus, beliefs, and intentions guide us toward manifesting these desired states in the field of pure health potentiality.

The Law of Empowered Perspective can be summarized as follows: "Optimum mindfulness and consideration of our habitual thinking, whether related to health or any other challenge, leads to optimum thought." Increasing our awareness and mindfulness of our desired health outcomes will improve our health. There is no better way to cultivate mindful awareness than by using an optimized Medical Mastermind approach.

* * *

The Think and Live Longer Mind Shift Hack:
Shifting Perspectives

In the movie "The Mask," starring Jim Carey, a mystical mask imbued with powers falls into the hands of an introverted bank teller, granting him supernatural abilities and transforming him into an outgoing and confident character. Inspired by his newfound persona, he exclaims, *"Somebody stop me!"* as he prepares to embark on an evening to pursue his love interest. This exclamation signifies his unwavering belief in his success and his determination to overcome any obstacles that may come his way.

Similarly, the following exercise focuses on your health challenge and on creating a successful health image. It aims to cultivate a profound, mindful awareness of your ultimate goal and your ability to achieve it. When evaluating your thoughts, say, *"Somebody stop me!"* Then, ask yourself the following questions:

WHAT DO I WANT?

WHY DO I WANT IT?

WHAT AM I WILLING TO GIVE TO RECEIVE IT?

This Socratic approach serves several purposes:

It helps you focus on the specific challenge or intention at hand while also establishing your expected outcomes and the actions you believe are necessary to achieve them.

Exploring your motivations for pursuing success in your current health challenge (or any other area) helps you tap into the emotions associated with your desired outcome.

It enables you to visualize and plan the pathways to potential success and consider the necessary information and potential setbacks along the way.

If you cannot envision a clear path toward your desired outcome, it may indicate the need to seek guidance from your Medical Mastermind or continue your research.

Now, take a moment to fill in the blanks below and align them with your current health optimization goal. Repeat and remind yourself of these statements as often as needed to stay focused on your goal:

I WANT:

BECAUSE:

I AM WILLING TO GIVE TO RECEIVE IT.

The Infinite Law of Supply in Health

*Within your subconscious depths lie infinite wisdom,
infinite power,
and an infinite supply of all that is necessary.* - Joseph
Murphy

Natalie, a thirty-nine-year-old obese woman, came to see me accompanied by her sister. She was a cancer survivor who had undergone a bone marrow transplant for acute leukemia eleven years ago, which led to various health issues, including chronic conjunctivitis, hypothyroidism, and arthritis. Before seeking my help, she was being treated for chronic pain, depression, and anxiety with multiple medications, including antidepressants, anti-anxiety drugs, and narcotic painkillers. Her mental health was further affected by the recent murder-suicide of her mother by her stepfather.

Natalie's main concerns centered around weight loss, hormonal balance, insomnia, anxiety, and depression. Although she had previously tried hormonal balancing with non-bioidentical hormones prescribed by her previous physician, she didn't experience any noticeable improvement. Her depression and anxiety were being managed with a selective serotonin reuptake inhibitor (SSRI), resulting in significant weight gain.

Additionally, Natalie was a heavy smoker and had no intention of quitting until her sister intervened. Due to her previous unsuccessful treatment and her diminishing hope for improvement, her sister's intervention became a turning point.

Upon evaluation, it was revealed that Natalie had insufficient levels of various hormones, including estradiol, testosterone, thyroid, and progesterone. Her cholesterol levels, especially LDL (the "bad" cholesterol), were also high. However, her blood work was normal, except for a mild macrocytic anemia.

Natalie's loss of hope had deeply impacted her. She couldn't envision any improvements in her situation until we discussed her goals for positive outcomes. As part of her optimization program, we employed a key technique to reinforce her success: creating an image of ideal health and well-being. She was instructed to focus on this desired image and update it as she saw fit throughout her treatment. This image was incorporated into guided meditation sessions assisted by brainwave entrainment technology. Natalie created her initial image shortly after her preliminary evaluations and has revisited and refined it multiple times. Supported by exercises like intention boards, her envisioned outcome now centers on a vibrant, active young woman wearing size eight clothing (down from her initial size of sixteen), who no longer smokes and is actively engaged with her social contacts and community.

While it is still early to make definitive conclusions, Natalie shows great promise in manifesting her desired self. She has quit smoking and has achieved 25% of her weight-loss goal. Her response to bioidentical hormone replacement therapy and supplementation has been positive, allowing her to discontinue SSRI medication. Her overall demeanor has become more positive, and her focus is firmly fixed on her envisioned goals.

In our discussions with patients, we use the law of supply to empower them to choose their desired health outcomes. This is integrated into imaging sessions using brainwave entrainment technology, which we recommend twice daily—morning and evening. These sessions reinforce the thought process that sustains ongoing motivation to achieve the envisioned goals. This approach is reminiscent of Napoleon Hill's influential book on success, "Think and Grow Rich," which has guided countless individuals in the business world.

The Law of Supply teaches us that whatever we desire and genuinely believe in our hearts is already ours. The fact that we have the desire and belief is evidence of the cause already existing. The cause is that our desire is already available to us when we feel the need or want. Our desired outcome is accessible because of our sincere desire, and will be provided to us accordingly.

The key to understanding the Law of Supply lies in our belief in the existence of what we desire. This is crucial because there is an unlimited supply of every good we can conceive of. We continuously utilize this law and have the right to a complete and ever-increasing supply of anything we want or need. It will be so as long as we believe in the outcome, maintain our desire, and expect it to manifest in our lives. The universal Law of Supply informs us that the fundamental substance of every conceivable good already exists, and our desires, thoughts, and images indicate that this good, stemming from the fundamental substance (the principle of quantum entanglement), is already within our reach.

In the Bible, Jesus said, *"Ask, and it shall be given to you; seek, and ye shall find; knock, and it shall be opened unto you"* (Matthew 7:7 KJV). This passage conveys that believing in the desired results is equivalent to achieving them. It also reminds us that we are not meant to settle for our current life circumstances. This doesn't mean we should be frustrated with our circumstances, though that can happen when we misunderstand the nature of challenges and obstacles. Instead, we are constantly progressing toward new states of enlightenment, knowledge, and physical being, offering fresh perspectives on our lives. From these perspectives, we develop new desires and better goals and outcomes. Jesus also said, *"What things soever ye desire, when ye pray, believe that ye receive them, and ye shall have them"* (Mark 11:24 KJV).

We can have reasonable confidence in the desired outcome because it already exists. It exists in our future as we have envisioned it: *"Believe it, then you will see it"* (though the same principle applies to adverse outcomes if we focus on the negative!). The supply is always ready and available to us.

Whatever we want is there for us; it cannot be any other way.

We should expect no less regarding our health, regardless of the perceived gap between our current state and where we want to be. Good health is available to us in abundance when we recognize the need for better health. We can access this supply simply by believing in and earnestly intending its presence in our lives. (Remember Fran?)

The active thought of our desire, the belief in improved health, is evidence that the supply exists. Our inspired idea for better physical, mental, and emotional well-being proves that the material supply is in our future. However, we must create the demand. Unfortunately, in most cases, we are unaware that we control the mechanism that always supplies it. This misconception is our downfall. Our thoughts are the architects of our health, and we must regard them as such.

Similarly, to our detriment, many trusted advisors and health-care professionals tend to focus on negative, undesirable outcomes. This approach is often adopted to prevent disappointment if the outcome is adverse. However, in a context of scarcity and fear, this advice is counterproductive, especially when it comes to creating quantum reality. It hinders our ability to construct a positive image of our desires.

At the outset, let us realize that the material world in which we live is a sphere of effects and that behind these effects is a world of causes.
Then recognize that when you desire any particular effect, it is because that [this] specific "good" is already in existence in the

sphere of causes.
Then recognize that when you desire any particular effect,
this desire is an appearance [in your consciousness] of an
underlying cause.
—Raymond Holliwell

As long as our thoughts focus on creating the desired outcome rather than the undesired one, the supply has already been generated and will flow toward that outcome. It is crucial not to lose sight of or weaken our connection to a healthy and positive image by getting distracted by worries or doubts about the outcome. If such thoughts arise, acknowledge them without judgment and redirect your focus to the desired outcome. Relaxation and confidence in the ultimate result are necessary to access the supply effectively. This relaxation and focus are part of the methodology used during morning and evening imaging sessions, supported by brainwave entrainment and guided imagery. These sessions transform our thoughts and minds into magnets for the optimal outcome we seek.

When our thoughts are consistently fixated on sickness and disease, we inadvertently prepare for and demand more sickness from the infinite supply. For example, let's focus on organizing and managing our medications for our illnesses. The universe responds by providing more of that experience: "Since you're so focused on caring for disease, we can certainly give you more of it!" Dwelling on thoughts like "my pain," "my swelling," "my weight," "my congestive heart failure," "my smoking," or any other negative self-identifications will only diminish the focus on demanding good from the infinite supply. That's why our focus must always be directed toward the best possible outcome we can envision. This mindset, along with each small success, will lead to new perspectives on incremental improvement and even better outcomes.

We must disregard the negative self-talk and discouraging thoughts of skeptics or those who constantly dwell on disease or adverse outcomes, regardless of the cost. Mind-body training programs, as do biofeedback technologies, offer techniques to shift our focus from negative to positive.

Remember, focused thoughts on our ideal outcome activate the infinite supply (the observer effect) and, subconsciously, stimulate the body's organs to improve our health. If you are overwhelmed by destructive thoughts, take a meditation break and recommit to positive imaging. Reflect on your accomplishments and cultivate gratitude. This will give you a clearer perspective on your progress and reinforce the knowledge that you are achieving your ideal. Additionally, using biofeedback or other mindfulness tools can help reorient our focus before negative thoughts gain enough momentum to lead to undesirable outcomes.

When we genuinely desire better health in any form or domain, it is because the desired end result of good health already exists for us. Although this may seem counterintuitive, it aligns with scientific principles formulated by renowned physicists in the early twentieth century—Einstein, Planck, Schrödinger, Bohr, and Heisenberg—who were Nobel laureates in physics (except for Everett).

The discoveries and theories of Einstein, Planck, Schrödinger,

Bohr, Heisenberg, and other scientists led to a paradigm shift in understanding the influence of thought on matter. They demonstrated that we are not mere observers of the material world, including our health, but active participants in shaping the outcomes and influencing the fabric of our universe and lives. This concept, however, is not entirely new. Religious and philosophical leaders have long recognized the impact of our thoughts and beliefs on our surroundings. We have just encountered quotes from the New Testament and from authors who predated the Nobel laureate physicists who established the principles of quantum physics. This understanding has existed for millennia, and only a few thousand years have passed since the scientific community provided empirical evidence that aligns with our intuitive insights.

The act of us simply looking at our world—
projecting the feelings and beliefs that we have as we
focus our awareness on the particles that the universe is
made of— changes those particles as we are looking.
—Gregg Braden, Author of The Spontaneous
Healing of Belief

In 1957, Hugh Everett III presented his doctoral thesis at Princeton, which addressed certain issues in quantum physics. His work introduced the scientific explanation of infinite parallel timelines and universes, known as the many-worlds interpretation of quantum mechanics. According to this interpretation, multiple past and future timelines exist alongside the present, and the differences among them are determined by the decisions we make and by our thoughts and beliefs at the time.

Additionally, the principle of quantum entanglement explains how actions on one seemingly independent object can affect another without direct contact, as Einstein famously called it "spooky action at a distance." This implies that one body can perceive the influence exerted on another without any physical connection. The many-worlds interpretation and quantum entanglement shed light on the universal Law of Supply, suggesting that our desired health image exists in a parallel future reality and that we desire its manifestation in our present health.

Pursuing empowered health implies that any desired outcome is possible once we believe it can be achieved. While the most effective approaches for improving our systems are still being explored and will depend on our unique genetic makeup, the modalities we are currently pursuing within the context of an empowered medicine program are proving effective, especially for managing chronic diseases. By aligning with the quantum nature of the universal laws and the principles of quantum physics, we are enhancing the effectiveness of conventional medicine. These quantum concepts were even discussed by Jesus in his teachings, as exemplified by his statement, *"Blessed are those who have not seen and yet have believed"* (John 20:29, New International Version).

This implies that the blessings of belief can be obtained without visualization. We will experience and obtain what we believe in—fulfilling our desires. Hence, quantum mechanics was discussed in the first century AD.

As we consciously choose to create a life of empowered health, our vision, mental imagery, and thoughts become the tools and driving force that guide us toward the desired outcome. In a quantum sense, we, as observers, shape our health by our fundamental beliefs and sustained focus on the desired outcome. Our thoughts manifest as the energy that ultimately shapes the image of excellent health we aspire to achieve.

* * *

The Think and Live Longer Mind Shift Hack: Creating Your Successful Health Image & Life Intention Board

Practicing visualization and setting intentions are two of the most powerful mind exercises we can do. According to Rhonda Byrne's popular book, "The Secret," the law of attraction forms our entire life experience through our core beliefs, thoughts, and feelings, whether we are conscious of it or not. When we visualize, we emit a powerful vibratory frequency that brings us whatever we focus on.

Combining visualization with intention setting is a proven process that helps us manifest our desires. In a quantum sense, it connects our entangled sense of future health success with our present-day health consciousness. Olympic athletes also use this process because it enhances their performance. Psychology Today reports that the brain patterns activated when a weightlifter physically lifts heavy weights are similarly activated when the lifter imagines (visualizes) lifting the weights.

To bring your desires to life, create a sacred space that represents them. Your energy flows where your attention goes, so placing an intention or vision board in a prominent location engages you in mini-visualization throughout the day.

There is no right or wrong way to create your intention board. The goal is to gather images and words that inspire you and help you maintain focus on your vision of an optimized, infinitely healthy body and life. When selecting images, choose ones that resonate with your highest vision. They should evoke positive emotions and represent the aspects you desire for your health and life.

For instance, if you dream of a home with a bedroom overlooking the ocean, select a picture of that home or the breathtaking view from the bedroom. Step into the picture and imagine waking up every morning to the sight of a crystal-clear blue ocean, a colorful sunrise, and the scent of salty air, all while staying in the comfort of your bed.

Similarly, for your vision of optimized health, you can choose a picture of someone else in an ideal state of health or of yourself at your healthiest. Step into that picture and imagine the abundance of energy, the profound sense of well-being, and the incredible adventures you will embark on when you achieve that perfect state of health.

Some people may struggle to identify what they desire for their lives. If you find yourself in that position, don't worry. It's perfectly okay. To gain clarity and start setting intentions for your infinite health and life, answer the following questions without overthinking the answers. Then ask yourself, "Now, what would be even better than that?" Push the boundaries of your imagination.

How would it look if you could have a life beyond your wildest imagination? Consider where you would live, who would be with you (or not), and what a typical day would entail. Think about the activities that bring you joy.

- How would you feel when you wake up in the morning?
- What practices, activities, or things could help you experience that feeling daily?
- When you were a child, what did you aspire to be when you grew up?
- Why did that dream captivate you?
- Is there anything you can do now that evokes the same sense of passion and excitement?

You intuitively understand what resonates with you and what doesn't. Trust your feelings as you select the pictures and quotes for your intention board. Here are a few quotes that I find inspiring:

"The secret to having it all is believing that you already

do." - Source unknown

"Our intention creates our reality." - Dr. Wayne Dyer

"Create the highest grandest vision possible for your life because you become what you believe." - Oprah Winfrey

"Whatever you hold in your mind consistently is what you will experience in your life." - Anthony Robbins

"If you are working on something you really care about, you do not have to be pushed— the vision pulls you."
—Steve Jobs

Your Intention Board - Fast & Furious NOS Style

I (*LeNae*) must admit that my knowledge of NOS (Nitrous Oxide Systems) primarily comes from the Fast and the Furious film series. As I understand it, when the character Brian O'Connor pushes the red NOS button during a drag race, his car accelerates so rapidly that it almost gives him whiplash. Brian thoroughly enjoys this experience. Including intentional affirmations in your daily intention board practice while focusing on your internal emotional guidance system is akin to adding high-grade NOS to your car. It allows you to attract what you desire even faster.

Everything in the universe is composed of energy vibrating at different levels. Our thoughts, words, and emotions are also forms of energy vibrating at various frequencies. When we consciously choose to think positively, speak positively, and embrace feelings of happiness, joy, bliss, and love, regardless of our current life circumstances, we align ourselves with our heart's desires. This alignment paves the way for the manifestation of what we truly want.

Ideally, dedicate a few minutes each morning before getting out of bed and each evening before falling asleep to meditate on your intention board. Immerse yourself in the feelings associated with the symbols and images you selected to represent your desired life. During this practice, repeat affirmations that support your intentions. For instance, if you seek more energy and a healthier body, your intentional affirmations could include:

- I am deeply grateful for my abundant energy.
- My energy reserves are limitless.
- I am profoundly grateful for my current state of health, knowing that I am already healed and whole.

By thinking intentionally, guided by your intention board, you will begin to speak intentionally. These practices will contribute to a sense of lightness and joy, opening the door to manifesting your desires when they appear before you.

Once you have completed your intention board, I invite you to take a picture of it and share it with us on your social media page -tag us on Instagram @Your.Infinite.Health

The Infinite Law of Attraction in Health

Steven, a forty-nine-year-old obese male, sought an evaluation for persistent pain in his lower left leg. This pain resulted from a left hip fracture and a heel bone fracture from a previous car accident several years ago. The accident also led to severe degenerative disease in his left knee, which required a total knee replacement eight months before his initial visit.

In addition to his knee pain, Steven was a long-term smoker of thirty years, consuming one to one and a half packs of cigarettes daily. He also had mild to moderate chronic obstructive pulmonary disease, mild hypertension, fatigue, mild cognitive dysfunction, mood swings, irritability, decreased libido, erectile dysfunction, and seasonal allergies.

Despite regularly visiting his family physician, Steven's doctor refused to address his knee pain or discuss his other significant health issues. The physician prescribed only blood pressure medication and ignored Steven's requests for further evaluation. Consequently, the State of Louisiana classified Steven as disabled, preventing him from re-entering the workforce.

Steven came to our pain-healing program on the recommendation of another patient who had experienced significant improvements. (We prefer the term "pain-healing" over "pain management" because our focus is on resolving the pain and alleviating its causes and aggravators using effective therapeutic interventions rather than relying solely on medication and procedures for control.) However, Steven was only interested in obtaining pain medication for his knee when he came to see me and showed no interest in exploring alternative techniques.

During the initial evaluation, we discovered that Steven had significantly decreased testosterone levels, moderately decreased bone density, severe vitamin D deficiency, and biochemical markers indicating early adrenal dysfunction. Elevated inflammatory markers and estradiol levels showed a high risk for coronary artery disease. His obesity and pre-diabetic blood glucose levels likely contributed to the elevated inflammatory indices. We recommended the following approach for Steven:

- Aggressive nutritional lifestyle modifications;
- Progressive exercise regimen involving non-impact high-intensity interval aerobic and flexibility training;
- Hormonal and metabolic optimization, along with nu-

traceutical supplementation;
- Mind-body techniques, including "Think and Live Longer" coaching and biofeedback.

After four to six months, Steven experienced significant pain improvement and no longer required a cane or other supportive devices for walking. His pain medication was significantly reduced to using a single 10-milligram hydrocodone preparation two to four times a day as needed, with occasional muscle relaxants in the evenings. He also quit smoking within two months of starting the program. His moodiness, cognitive function, libido, energy levels, and endurance significantly improved with hormonal optimization. All metabolic, endocrine, and inflammatory parameters remained within optimum ranges throughout his treatment.

What I found most enlightening was Steven's unwavering focus and determination to improve once he realized it was possible. This mindset shift and the resulting improvements in his well-being are typical among my patients. Steven diligently followed the program's instructions and maintained a positive attitude, firmly believing his desired outcome was attainable.

The Law of Attraction can be summarized as "like attracts like." This concept suggests that our thoughts and desires, whether positive or negative, manifest corresponding experiences in our health and overall lives. Our thoughts are a form of energy, and these energetic desires and beliefs influence the attraction of similar energetic health outcomes.

In essence, the manifestation of favorable health outcomes depends on the power of our thought energy—our desires, intentions, and visions—to influence the underlying energy fields (such as the ether or quantum field of infinite potentiality). It's essential to recognize that our conceptual abilities, specifically our mind and executive brain function, enable us to imprint our intentions on the surrounding energy fields, effectively bringing about change and allowing us to reap the benefits of our creativity.

Understanding this concept is particularly relevant to our health because our bodies are constantly remodeling in response to our ideas, thoughts, intentions, and actions. For example, simply intending to quit smoking creates an entirely different epigenetic and intracellular environment, initiating the remodeling of subsequent cells generated from the existing ones. Considering that our body's cells regenerate entirely over about seven years (depending on the organ), we can easily see the impact of our intent to attract excellent health (such as improving breathing and preventing smoking-related lung disease) or not. It's fascinating to note that the Law of Attraction has ancient philosophical roots and is supported by current findings in quantum physics, as briefly discussed in the chapter on the Law of Supply. The concept was embraced in the 1800s by New Thought philosopher and healer Phineas Quimby, who apparently "healed" himself of tuberculosis despite multiple failed medical treatments. Quimby's mind-body approach gained significant popularity, particularly in conjunction with hypnotism.

New Thought authors and healers attributed many "dis-eases"

to negative emotional thought processes such as fear, lack, worry, stress, and other negative thinking patterns. They also believed that healing and well-being resulted from positive or "right" thoughts.

This "new thinking" philosophy extends beyond health and disease prevention to encompass wealth, relationships, and success across various domains. The same principle underlies concepts presented in "Think and Grow Rich," one of the best-selling personal development and business references ever.

"Whatever the mind can conceive and believe, it can achieve." —Napoleon Hill

If you desire something related to your health, it already exists. Your desire must be paired with expectation (intent) to achieve the outcome you expect.

"Always rid yourself of desires in order to observe its secrets, but always allow yourself to have desires in order to observe its manifestations."
—Lao Tzu, Tao Te Ching

This means we experience a sense of completeness and wholeness when free from desires. However, desires are what lead to manifestations. Therefore, if we can master our focus and attention in the present moment, we can define and expect what we want to manifest and attract into our lives. From an individual perspective, this means that by desiring and intending good health, we can manifest good for ourselves and the benefit of all.

Desire is a focused interest or longing for something. Our empowered intentions for excellent health are supported by our desires, which fuel and reinforce them. If excellent health is defined uniformly within a population, individuals must draw greater attention to their desired outcomes and infuse them with their unique qualities. We must consistently and effectively direct our desire toward our intent through ongoing effort.

Unfortunately, many people with chronic health issues become consumed by thoughts of their disease. Their daily lives revolve around medication delivery and activities that do not improve their health. This type of focus leads to repeated actions and habits detrimental to their well-being. The expectation and intention of maintaining good health no longer enter their thinking, and they have no interest in focusing on it because of the overwhelming need to manage various aspects of their condition. For example, I encounter pain-healing patients like Steven who solely focus on their pain medication and refer to their pain or illness as if it were a cherished pet. In this context, the quantum perspective suggests that neither the focused thoughts nor the emotional energy required to transform the field of pure potentiality into material reality are present. In other words, they are not using the Law of Attraction to improve their health.

Another example is a diabetic individual focusing solely on high blood sugar levels and the prescription medications needed to control them. These individuals would be better served by focusing on comfort, ease of function, and optimal nutrient processing.

When we examine our current healthcare system and its reactive approach to care, we observe that most treatments focus on quick prescription delivery and symptom management rather than comprehensive, long-term problem resolution. Only when physicians are genuinely interested in healing and facilitating excellent health and its acquisition will we begin to witness positive changes. If healthcare providers no longer expect to see resolution and instead lack the desire to treat, the intent to cure, or the appropriate compassion to facilitate true healing, it becomes challenging for patients to focus on resolving their medical challenges.

How can the "trusting uneducated" alter the deeply ingrained thoughts that have become the collective standard of care? A prime example of this is the current issue of pain "management." If we focus solely on managing pain, we lose interest in resolving it.

Expectation, belief, and intent play crucial roles in the Law of Attraction. Expectation and intent are active forms of belief in an outcome. Expectation is the strong belief that something will happen in the future, accompanied by the feeling of hope and the belief in ultimate achievement or intent. Desire connects us to the health we want, directing our attention to the outcome. Expectation, which generates forward momentum, draws that desired health towards us.

The Sequencing Formula for an Empowered Health Destiny:

Thought and thinking lead to beliefs and actions. And these actions become habits when repeated; they also reinforce the beliefs, which lead to new habits, which lead to new character traits and destiny! The new thoughts and insights gained through our independent education, along with the information and mentorship provided by our Medical Mastermind, will help us form new, well-founded beliefs and actions. The actions necessary to attract this new health outcome are those actions that we take of our own volition, as well as those that our Mastermind may guide or empower us to effectuate. With or without prescription medication, this guidance is the active component that further reinforces or optimizes the connection (attraction) with the imagined empowered health outcome we desire (destiny).

Desire is closely tied to expectation, and expecting something leads to its achievement. This principle is important for our health. Working with our Mastermind, we visualize our recoveries from chronic diseases. Our positive expectations pave the way for triumph. However, if we desire an athlete's physical fitness and health but do not expect to attain them, we are merely dreaming without anticipating our desires. When our empowered actions align with our beliefs, we attract and fulfill our empowered health destiny.

One essential action we are already taking is creating the mental image of our desired health outcome through the twice-daily brainwave entrainment meditations. This practice resembles the techniques employed by professional athletes to achieve peak performance in competition. We are dedicated to training for optimal health and longevity. Consider the biblical narrative in 2 Kings 4:1–7, where a widow approached the prophet Elisha seeking help because she was in debt and her sons were at risk of becoming slaves. Elisha asked her what she had in her house, and she said she had only a small pot of extra lamp oil. Elisha instructed her to borrow empty vessels from her neighbors, emphasizing that she should borrow many. Once she had gathered the vessels, she would go inside, close the door, and pour the oil into each one. She followed his instructions, and the oil miraculously flowed until all the vessels were filled. When she informed Elisha that she had completed the task, he advised her to sell the oil, pay her debts, and live on the remaining funds. This story illustrates the concept of receiving what we expect. It encourages us to push the limits of our imagination and embrace the possibilities ahead.

* * *

The Think and Live Longer Mindset Hack: Intention Boarding - The Next Level

In the previous chapters, you started your daily meditation practice and created your Successful Health and Life Intention Board. You've also been dedicating at least ten to fifteen minutes each day to focus on the symbols and representations of your desired optimal health and life, fully immersing yourself in the feeling of already having it. Great job on your progress! Now, let's take your intention to focus to the next level.

Over the next few weeks, choose one to two items from your intention board and actively seek out references to them throughout your day. For instance, if you aspire to participate in a marathon, start noticing runners and running-related things in your surroundings. It could be someone jogging along the roadside, conversations about running happening around you, or even running scenes on television. Another example could be if you have the word "joy" on your intention board. Begin to notice every occurrence of the word "joy" during your day. It might be meeting someone named Joy, spotting the word on a billboard, or coming across it in a magazine.

This mind-shift hack demonstrates that energy flows to where our attention goes. By consciously shifting our focus toward what we desire, we begin to attract those experiences into our lives, whether in health, relationships, or wealth. Remember to keep it light-hearted. Approach it as a game you play with yourself, and you can even involve your partner and/or children to join in on the fun.

The Infinite Law of Receiving in Health

Roger, a thirty-eight-year-old dedicated to his health, has been a patient partner for several years. While he doesn't have many medical issues, he recently faced challenges related to his desire to win a bodybuilding competition. Despite his efforts, he was frustrated by his inability to achieve the desired muscle definition and lower body fat levels necessary for competitive success. This was a new experience for him since he had previously seen improvements in his physique through increased effort at the gym. However, his motivation and ability declined over the past year, and he no longer aligned with his vision.

Apart from a slightly more noticeable fat layer during his physical examination, Roger didn't exhibit any remarkable findings. However, his lab results showed lower levels of certain hormones and nutrients, which may affect his overall well-being. We addressed these sub-optimal levels to help him regain focus and motivation. In the following weeks, he experienced a significant improvement in his sense of well-being, which fueled his ability to concentrate on his goals. He went beyond his usual efforts, and before the competition, during his final follow-up, he shared that he had already made space on his trophy wall for his anticipated victory.

The Infinite Law of Receiving can be summarized as follows: *"To receive the best in proportion to what you give, you must give your best."* It's another universal law that requires multiple actions to fully benefit from it. To harness this law effectively, it's crucial to understand our position within the universal energy field. This field responds to our desires and beliefs, enabling us to create whatever we want in life. The practical outcome of applying the infinite laws to our lives is the manifestation of our desires. Suppose the Infinite Law of Supply (quantum entanglement and multiple worlds) has generated our desire for something, and our intention and expectation (Law of Attraction) draw us closer to that desired outcome. In that case, the Infinite Law of Receiving determines the conditions of receiving based on our alignment with the universal energy of creation and supply (the limitless potential of the quantum field).

Like all basic principles in the universe, this law is founded on the energetic equilibrium that exists between all things, because all material things are energy ($E{=}{=}mc2$). We are therefore striking an energetic equilibrium with our supplier of good (energy). It is the dynamic parity required before any energy exchange can occur, in any form, and it includes our optimized health. As Jesus said,

*"Give and it shall be given unto you: good measure,
pressed down, shaken together, and running over will be
put into thy bosom. For with the same measure that you
use,
it will be measured back to you." - Luke 6:38 - NKJV*

Let's examine this equilibrium from an unbiased observer's perspective, which allows us to view it from both the recipient's and the donor's perspectives simultaneously. When we receive, we are also giving. So we can interpret the passage as "I have given, and it is given unto me." Since all material goods are created from source (quantum) energy, it's a matter of perspective. Moreover, the more we work with this energetic equilibrium, the more it works for us. It's like receiving a generous portion that overflows and abundantly fills our lives. Essentially, we are giving and receiving from ourselves at the same time. This spiritual principle aligns with the law of energy conservation in physics, which states that the quality of the energy we receive equals the energy we give.

This principle holds true for our health. We all desire optimal health, which is essential for a fulfilling life. However, when we consider something we desire, such as good health, we often think we must receive it before we can give it. This mindset reveals a lack of understanding of how the law works. To maintain the crucial energetic equilibrium, we must begin by giving before we can receive.

As expressed in Luke 6:38, giving is fundamental to creating from the source of energy. If our focus remains solely on "getting" good health, with a limited perspective, it's unlikely that we will achieve and experience the best health possible. This mindset is akin to thinking that extraordinary health can be achieved simply by taking a pill. However, defining extraordinary health and considering the pill's capabilities may alter this perspective. Personally, I envision extraordinary health as a happy child at play, and I doubt it can be achieved through medication alone.

The Law of Receiving. gratitude forrequires giving before receiving, similar to the idea of praying blessings. Creating a prayer of gratitude or a mental image of our desired health elevates our vibrational energy. This energy strengthens the entangled communication we emit and connects us to a parallel or future quantum existence where our desired health already exists. This is the quantum system on which we impose our beliefs. As this vibration is emitted outward, binding us and helping us receive our desired supply, we need to relax and prepare to receive its benefits. In essence, our intention to achieve optimum health transmits the vibration of expectant belief to our desired future, resulting in the observer effect of materialization. Following this transmission, which is the driving force, and depending on the intensity of the emitted vibration, we receive the desired improvements or upgrades.

From a physics perspective, we need to understand entangled communication a little better. This communication occurs between two bodies vibrating at similar, if not identical, frequencies. It is unlikely to be functional between vibrational bodies with highly different frequencies. Recognizing this caveat is essential and will be clarified in the Law of Increase.

From a molecular biological standpoint, what impact does this have on how our system operates? As we discussed earlier, our thoughts, beliefs, and past actions have shaped our current health. It's time to acknowledge the thoughts and beliefs that influence certain epigenetic expressions of our genes, both beneficial and detrimental, which ultimately determine the state of our bodies today. By following the guidance in this book, we are actively modifying our thoughts, beliefs, and expressions, leading us toward our chosen healthy future.

There are infinite possibilities for health outcomes, and countless timelines we can traverse to reach them. With our newfound knowledge and abilities, we can achieve any desired image. This is the foundation of these laws. Our thoughts and their vibrations reach out systematically, connecting us to our desired future health. Using these laws helps us stay connected and bring that future closer.

I have often heard patient partners, even those in their thirties, express the belief that they are too old to make a change. This consideration should not apply to anyone. We learn to read when we can barely run across a schoolyard during the first five years of our lives. I may understand this attitude more from a ninety-year-old with multiple end-of-life organ failures and compromised health. The truth is that, regardless of age or physical condition, we are capable of miraculous change and of undertaking endeavors. We create our reality in every given moment. This interpretation aligns with the concept of biocentrism and our quantum reality. We need only create an image of what we want, which becomes ours. This is the Law of Supply.

What role does giving play in the Law of Receiving? Giving is intertwined with our envisioned health outcomes. We create images of excellent blood pressure, optimal blood sugar metabolism, and a healthy skeletal structure through our imagination. In this imagined intent, we generate a vibration that matches the intensity of our desire to receive. This vibration is sent out, and if our vibrational self is aligned, prepared, and receptive, we will receive the supply of optimized health.

However, there are a few key points to clarify about receiving. When we perceive that we lack the optimal health we desire, it stems from a sense of deprivation. This can be a perception of having previously had good health and now lacking it, or of never having had good health at all. Deprivation and lack are disempowered states of being associated with low-vibrational emotions such as anger, craving, fear, anxiety, grief, regret, despair, guilt, and shame. These emotions are often linked to poor or declining health.

On the other hand, good health resides in a state of possession, an empowered state of being. Empowered states of being are characterized by emotions such as gratitude, satisfaction, optimism, hopefulness, forgiveness, acceptance, love, serenity, joy, bliss, and enlightenment. The serene, relaxed state that accompanies these states of consciousness has been associated with spontaneous healing, enhanced cellular repair mechanisms, and improved metabolism.

Therefore, when we imagine our optimized health, it is crucial to do so from an empowered state. Instead of "asking" for optimized health from a place of lack or deprivation, we must understand and embody the Law of Supply, which states that what we desire is already ours. Our optimized health is already within our grasp. Ideally, we should express gratitude in advance, having faith that our optimized health is coming to fruition. It's essential to understand the symbiotic relationship between giving and receiving. While many people associate giving with money, viewing it as a powerful entity that controls their lives, from a philosophical perspective, money is a form of energy that serves our purposes. It is an agent of energetic exchange that operates according to our intentions. It symbolizes the universal energy we engage with to manifest our desires and respond to our will. If giving always precedes receiving, it is through our thoughts (which lead to actions and beliefs), our words (derived from our thoughts), and our actions and service (directed towards ourselves or others) that we align with the law and manifest the positive outcomes we desire or intend.

I mention money not because it directly relates to achieving our ultimate health goal, but because our thoughts about money can reveal our understanding (or misunderstanding) of giving and receiving.

Let's take a moment to consider this. Giving of ourselves involves the effort of preparing ourselves to receive the benefits of abundance that we already possess, whether it's financial abundance or improved health. Take the example of Roger. We give effort through:

- **Thoughts:** This includes thinking about new mental activities like guided meditations or energy healing, as well as new physical activities such as low-impact exercising, yoga, or tai chi. It also involves exploring new spiritual activities. We may have been advised to find new recipes to achieve our nutritional goals. As discussed earlier regarding the Law of Thinking, this also involves consistently imagining and meditating on our ultimate health outcome. By thinking these thoughts, we connect with the supply and acknowledge the power of thought to transform our health into the desired image.

- **Words:** Using only positive health affirmations in our speech is essential. Even if someone like Gregg's mother has told us that we have always been and will always be a sickly child, we need to avoid negative affirmations.

> *"A fool's mouth is his destruction, and his lips are the snare of his soul."*
> - Proverbs 18:7

> *"A man's belly shall be satisfied with the fruit of his mouth; and with the increase of his lips shall he be filled. Death and life are in the power of the tongue; and they that love it shall eat the fruit thereof."* - Proverbs 18:20, 21

- **Actions:** This involves taking decisive action on our exercise plans, nutritional plans, and mind-body exercises like meditation or HeartMath training. It includes actively engaging in disciplines that promote health.

"However many holy words you read, however many you speak, what good will they do you if you do not act upon them?" - Buddha

- **Beliefs:** Beliefs are personal assumptions of truth that can either benefit or detrimentally affect our well-being and health. Whether these beliefs are objectively true or false is not as significant as their impact on our well-being. For example, a sugar pill can bring about improvement if one believes in its potency, just as a false negative assumption can lead to deterioration. Identifying negative assumptions and actively seeking truthful, verifiable information are important for addressing our specific issues. This process involves asking "why" and taking personal responsibility for finding answers. The Medical Mastermind alliance plays a crucial role in this process, which is essential for achieving our ultimate health outcomes.

Remember, the Law of Supply ultimately leads to physical and biomolecular changes that determine our new health outcomes, and these outcomes can be whatever we desire. Our beliefs allow these outcomes to manifest in our physical reality.

It's important to note that beliefs operate at the subconscious level. Our subconscious minds cannot correct erroneous notions. If we say, "I can't do something," our subconscious minds will work to ensure we can't. Conversely, if we say, "I can do something," "I am something," "I have something," our subconscious minds will work to bring those thoughts and beliefs into reality just as effectively. This is why it is crucial to always believe in our capabilities. Through conditioning of our subconscious and the activation of genetic variability via epigenetic mechanisms, our unconscious metabolism is driving positive changes in our body's environment.

The next aspect of the Law of Receiving is preparing to receive. When we prepare to receive, we actively believe and expect that our requests will be met with the desired response or resolution. As we have imagined a specific outcome for our health-related issue, the Law of Supply ensures it will manifest in our future. Preparing to receive also aligns with the Law of Thinking, which states that what we believe, we eventually see. It involves demonstrating faith and expectation, as discussed in the Law of Attraction.

A fun example for those on weight-optimization programs is engaging in anticipatory shopping for new dresses or pants that will fit their future bodies. For individuals pursuing incremental physical conditioning, this may involve signing up for programs in advance that require greater fitness than their current level. These actions demonstrate active faith and belief in realizing our desired health image. They help keep the image of success and intent alive and energize the power of reception. By establishing subconscious performance optimization, we create the conditions for quantum input that generate epigenetic changes, leading to optimized, healthy genetic expression.

However, we should also be cautious of the opposite situation that may arise from underlying limiting beliefs. These beliefs can lead to harmful behavior or character traits. Referring back to Proverbs 12:14, "A man shall be satisfied with good by the fruit of his mouth," and the teachings of Florence Shinn, if we ask for success but prepare for failure, we will indeed receive the situation we have prepared for. We should not ask for success while expecting the worst or preparing for the worst. If we do so, we will attract and receive exactly that. Expecting failure or feeling we won't succeed will lead us down that path.

> *"Argue for your limitations, and sure enough, they're yours."*
> - Richard Bach, author of Jonathan Livingston Seagull

Acts of preparing to receive engage our heartfelt emotions and intentions. They help eliminate doubt, fear, and other emotions that hinder reception or diminish our vibrational energy. Our expectations of good health increase as we strengthen the connection to the expected image of success. The strength of applying these simple and proven principles determines the quality of our outcomes. We become the guide to the quality of the outcome through the attributes of our preparation. If the energy of receiving is scalable, then the force and power of our preparations to receive excellent health through any action become the key to our success.

* * *

The Think and Live Longer Mind Shift Hack: Setting Yourself Up for Success in the Morning

"What you want will come after you have first given of yourself."
—Trip Goolsby, MD

Taking proactive, deliberate steps to set yourself up for a successful morning is crucial for a productive day. Assuming you have been diligent and consistent with the previous Think and Live Longer Mindset Hacks, this Mindset Hack builds upon your previous efforts.

Once you've completed your morning meditation, you can integrate this practice into your daily routine while brushing your teeth, showering, or enjoying your morning coffee. Ask yourself, "What is one new action I am committed to taking today to achieve my optimized health and longevity?"

Your answer could be as simple as drinking more water and reducing alcohol consumption, or choosing to take the stairs instead of the elevator. It might involve fully embracing the Think and Live Longer Mindset Hacks experientially, signing up for a local marathon, or even daring to skip the Starbucks line.

Remember, you become what you say you are and what you believe you are. Therefore, your self-talk must serve you positively. One effective way to shift your inner dialogue is to create and regularly repeat positive affirmations that support your successful health image (SHI). Here are some examples to help you get started:

- I am vital and energetic.
- I am calm and relaxed.
- I have my optimal body composition, and I maintain it.
- I am strong and flexible.
- I have a healthy mind.

If these affirmations don't feel entirely true to you, remember that you can approach them with gratitude and faith, as if you have already achieved them. According to the Law of Supply, they are already within your reach.

The Infinite Law of Increase in Health

"Once you make a decision, the universe conspires to make it happen."
— Ralph Waldo Emerson

The Christmas season has always been a bit stressful for me, as I often find myself caught up in the rush of Christmas Eve shopping. One particular season stands out in my memory, marked by a new refrigerator magnet with the words: *"Dear Santa, I want it all! I want it now! And I want it delivered!"* This quote often comes to mind when I first evaluate my patients and consider their desires and expectations. We all want to achieve optimal health and recovery as soon as possible. This is where the Law of Increase comes into play.

The principle of the Law of Increase is to enhance, amplify, strengthen, or accelerate the manifestation of our desired health outcomes. Understanding this simple principle will help you resolve many chronic medical issues and keep your mind focused on positive outcomes. Praise and gratitude are the pathways through which this universal law operates.

In my practice, I incorporate maintaining a gratitude journal as part of patient care. Consistently keeping a gratitude journal allows us to express practical thankfulness and encourages us to delve deeper into our relationship with the Source. According to Raymond Holliwell, when we praise or express gratitude to God for the things we desire, *"the fulfillment of that desire is accelerated to almost magical proportions."*

Praise and gratitude hold great significance. We can only receive those things, such as optimal health and financial abundance, that we desire from the source of supply, coupled with the belief and expectation of receiving them. Remember that asking or pleading does not reflect an expectant posture. As we discussed earlier, quantum entanglement and the vibrational energy of lack are not aligned with the act of possessing what we desire. There is no sense of expectation when we beg for charity. Our expectant attitude should be one of affirmation, declaration, assertive thanksgiving, and gratitude for having already received what has been created for us. This means that our successful health image is already ours, and we expedite its manifestation through grateful thanksgiving. Gratitude, defined by faith and expectancy, becomes the primary catalyst for the universal benefits we seek.

In Mark 11:24, Jesus says, *"What things soever ye desire, when ye pray, believe that ye receive them, and ye shall have them"* (KJV). The Law of Increase states that the expectant gratitude for having received the outcomes of our desires enhances the likelihood of receiving them.

It's important to note that praise or gratitude does not affect God or the Source in any way. The impact of gratitude lies in how it aligns our desired supply with us and makes it available to us energetically. By raising our vibration to match that of improved health, which operates at a higher energy level than illness, we become receptive to our desired health outcome. Gratitude and the accompanying feelings carry a high vibrational energy. Gratitude places our conscious being on a higher plane of energy, allowing us to embrace the desired health outcome and draw it towards us.

This concept of consciously elevating our vibrational energy may require some clarification. David Hawkins, MD, Ph.D., correlated energy levels with different levels of consciousness and developed a consciousness scale, which we will explore shortly. The concept of vibrational energy levels of all forms of matter and life was postulated by Egyptian philosophers around 5,000 BC. We are all composed of atoms, elements, and the biological substances that arise from their combinations. Each atom and subatomic particle has an optimal vibrational frequency that defines its element. Similarly, different molecules and proteins have different vibrational frequencies that define their structures in different states of matter, such as solid, liquid, and gas.

Water is a prime example of the importance of vibrational frequencies in our bodies. It constitutes approximately sixty to sixty-five percent of our total body weight. The vibrational frequencies of water can be measured and vary based on factors such as its physical state (solid, liquid, or gas) and atomic bonding angles. These frequencies are unique to each individual and are influenced by factors such as health, mood, stress levels, activity, ambient temperature, and more. Therefore, our emotional state and our ability to express gratitude offer simple ways to elevate our vibratory energy without resorting to extreme measures like boiling ourselves!

Water has also provided us with remarkable insights into how mood and emotions affect the physical body. Dr. Masaru Emoto conducted experiments analyzing the crystal structure of water exposed to various emotions, including love, hate, and gratitude. The findings were astonishing: positive emotions generated beautiful, organized, microscopic crystalline structures, while negative emotions caused the water to form disorganized, chaotic structures. This suggests that positive feelings, such as gratitude (which encompasses love and appreciation), are more likely to attract positive outcomes than negative emotions like fear, guilt, shame, and anger. Just imagine the profound effects of consistently practicing positive affirmations with a mindset of gratitude and, conversely, the detrimental effects of persistent negative self-talk.

Since our vibrational energy constantly changes from moment to moment, it can be challenging to monitor and control. Thankfully, we have tools at our disposal, such as the scale of consciousness developed by Dr. David R. Hawkins and presented in his book "Healing and Recovery." This scale, developed through Hawkins' extensive work in mindfulness and applied kinesiology, provides a practical way to intentionally shift our energy levels.

The Map of Consciousness

GOD-VIEW	LIFE-VIEW	LEVEL	LOG		EMOTION	PROCESS
Self	Is	Enlightenment	700-1000		Ineffable	Pure Consciousness
All-Being	Perfect	Peace	600	↑	Bliss	Illumination
One	Complete	Joy	540	↑	Serenity	Transfiguration
Loving	Benign	Love	500	↑	Reverence	Revelation
Wise	Meaningful	Reason	400	↑	Understanding	Abstraction
Merciful	Harmonious	Acceptance	350	↑	Forgiveness	Transcendence
Inspiring	Hopeful	Willingness	310	↑	Optimism	Intention
Enabling	Satisfactory	Neutrality	250	↑	Trust	Release
Permitting	Feasible	Courage	200	↑	Affirmation	Empowerment
Indifferent	Demanding	Pride	175	↓	Scorn	Inflation
Vengeful	Antagonistic	Anger	150	↓	Hate	Aggression
Denying	Disappointing	Desire	125	↓	Craving	Enslavement
Punitive	Frightening	Fear	100	↓	Anxiety	Withdrawal
Disdainful	Tragic	Grief	75	↓	Regret	Despondency
Condemning	Hopeless	Apathy	50	↓	Despair	Abdication
Vindictive	Evil	Guilt	30	↓	Blame	Destruction
Despising	Miserable	Shame	20	↓	Humiliation	Elimination

> ▓ The Final Doorway to Enlightenment/Nonduality
> ▓ The beginning of Integrity
> ▓ The beginning of the Nonlinear Realm

Notice the range of lower-vibrational emotions, such as humiliation, blame, despair, regret, anxiety, craving, hate, and scorn. By practicing motivational mindfulness techniques, we can become more aware of these emotions and strive to attain higher, less stressful vibrational levels. The higher our vibrational level, the faster we can access and affirm the improved health image we desire.

Even a gradual shift from a lower to a slightly higher vibrational level allows us to refine our subconscious goals and achieve increasingly positive outcomes. This is because our vibrational frequencies align with better results in well-being. By expressing gratitude and praise for the results we have already attained, we invite continuous improvement and can enhance our progress step by step.

On the other hand, complaints, criticism, despair, and anxious anticipation of outcomes lower our vibrational energy and hinder or delay our optimized health results. When we encounter occasional plateaus, it's important to remember this and return to gratitude for the progress we have already made, thereby recharging our vibrational energy. It's crucial to reassess our improvements and successes periodically, express gratitude for recent accomplishments, and be thankful for the future enhancements that await us.

Being grateful lifts our spirits, and the continued practice of gratitude fosters transformative attitudes that lead to even greater outcomes of greater benefit. Think of how, on each Thanksgiving Day, we are reminded to reflect upon each Thanksgiving and give thanks for what we have been blessed with. This is the same feeling we are to summon when raising our vibrational energy, except here we should focus on the good that lies ahead for us, not just on what has already transpired. This stalwart belief in the optimized health given to us in our image - even in the face of current challenges, be they multiple medical problems or results that seem to be in direct contradiction to what we want - that makes it come to pass. In other words, believing leads to seeing!

We achieve what we expect and anticipate. We achieve what we believe in and express gratitude for. This active form of belief, combined with heartfelt gratitude, raises our energy and creates a healing, rejuvenating environment throughout our bodies, affecting our hormones, metabolism, and immune system. It activates positive molecular pathways that promote epigenetic changes, ultimately transforming the foundation of our health.

In the context of chronic diseases, adopting the mindset of an "inverse paranoid" can be beneficial. It involves choosing to believe that the world is conspiring to bring us good. This mindset raises our awareness to the point of motivational or transitional change, and in doing so, our grateful awareness and conscious optimistic perception subtly transform us, preventing further deterioration of well-being and health. The key to health success lies in perceiving setbacks or illnesses as catalysts for achieving significantly better health in the near future.

"I operate as though everyone is part of a plot to enhance my well-being."
—Stan Dale, founder of the Human Awareness Institute

Our vibrational energy attracts improved health by maintaining a state of gratitude and positive expectation. This principle is likely a fundamental aspect of the successful Coué autosuggestion method, as exemplified by Emile Coué, a French pharmacist and psychologist in the late nineteenth century. Coué's patients, who consistently repeated the affirmation "Every day, in every way, I'm getting better and better," experienced fewer illnesses and setbacks than patients of other physicians at the time.

Raymond Holliwell succinctly captures the essence of gratitude in his quote: *"Be ever grateful for the very least of things, and the very most will come to you."* This reminder emphasizes the importance of cultivating gratitude even for minor successes or lifestyle modifications, such as losing one pound or adding one minute of exercise. Embracing gratitude positions us to attract incredible long-term benefits for our health outcomes.

* * *

The Think and Live Longer Mind Shift Hack: Practicing Gratitude

When our children were younger and attended the same school, we established a daily morning routine of expressing gratitude. We would list at least ten things we were grateful and thankful for each day. It became a fun game for the kids, competing to see who could list ten things the fastest. Over time, they even memorized their lists. However, what truly mattered was developing a consistent attitude of gratitude.

It's easy to take things and people for granted, especially during challenging and stressful times. However, it is precisely in those moments that cultivating a deliberate and mindful practice of gratitude becomes crucial.

Expressing gratitude and being thankful opens the door to receiving more of what we desire in our health and lives. Gratitude, often overlooked, is a secret superpower for those who regularly harness and apply it in their lives.

Gratitude is a state of being we achieve when we intentionally practice it, even when we don't feel grateful. It's okay if we don't always feel like we're "walking on sunshine" or experiencing constant joy. We can speak words of gratitude until we believe them.

Journaling is an excellent tool for cultivating a habit of gratitude. In the book's appendix, we have included a printable 14-Day gratitude journal. Each day, whether in the morning or evening, take a few minutes to thoughtfully consider and write down at least ten things you are thankful and grateful for. But don't stop there—go deeper. Explain why you are grateful for each person, place, thing, or event. Feel the emotions associated with your gratitude and repeat the words "Thank you, thank you, thank you."

By practicing this Mindset Hack every day for 14 days, you will begin to notice subtle shifts in the ease and grace of your day. Your desire to engage in behaviors that nourish your body, yourself, and others will begin to manifest. Consistency and authenticity are key as you establish a new habit of consciously practicing gratitude.

The Infinite Law of Compensation in Health

"To become the spectator of one's own life is to escape the suffering of life."
- Oscar Wilde

Rita, a forty-nine-year-old woman, came for an evaluation due to various health issues. She was obese and had diabetes, back pain, arthritis, hypertension, depression, anxiety, and mood instability. Her condition had not significantly improved despite seeking help from her primary internist and taking prescribed medications for hypertension and moodiness. She had not received hormone replacement therapy despite experiencing menopause three years ago. Rita had also noticed weight gain and worsening diabetes, requiring more insulin. Her main concern was the increasing back pain that limited her daily activities. To cope with anxiety and moodiness, she smoked fifteen to twenty cigarettes daily, a habit she had started in her twenties. She had a scaly rash and degenerative arthritic changes in her hands. Imaging and pulmonary function tests revealed bone density reduction, degenerative changes in the lumbar spine, and mild obstructive changes in her lung function.

After starting hormone replacement therapy and making lifestyle changes involving nutrition and exercise, Rita experienced significant improvements. Within three weeks of taking hormones, she no longer needed antidepressant medications, and within six weeks, she quit smoking without medication. After nine months, Rita reported increased energy and initiative, with no relapses into a melancholic state. Her commitment to self-investment and mind-body behavioral modification training transformed her attitude, replacing her previous focus on past failures and future dread with excitement and forward thinking.

While Rita's diabetes presented some challenges due to social issues and compliance concerns, her insulin therapy was eliminated within five months. At six and a half months, she no longer required prescription medications. Rita achieved substantial weight loss and continued to progress. Her elevated blood pressure, controlled with a single medication, was expected to improve further with ongoing efforts. Her arthritic symptoms and rash improved significantly, requiring only occasional over-the-counter anti-inflammatory medication. An energetic vision of a healthy future and a pain-free, active life replaced Rita's stress and resignation towards potential complications from diabetes and hypertension.

This case raises the question of effort-related compensation. To explore this concept, we need to understand the Law of Compensation, a compound law that considers the completion of seemingly competing polarities within the concept of universal wholeness, particularly in the acquisition of health and well-being.

> *"An inevitable dualism bisects nature so that each thing is half and suggests another thing to make it whole; as, spirit, matter; man, woman; odd, even; subjective, objective; in, out; upper, under; motion, rest; yea, nay. While the world is thus dual, so is every one of its parts."*
> —Ralph Waldo Emerson, Essays: First Series: Compensation (1841)

The polarities we observe in life are part of a continuous spectrum, and their significance depends on the viewer's perspective. As Emerson wrote in his essays, some leveling circumstances bring down the overbearing and fortunate individuals, placing them on the same ground as others. For instance, someone who is strong and fierce but lacks social skills may find humility and courtesy through their love and fear for their children.

This universal law compels us to acknowledge the importance of balance in every aspect of life, including our health. By striving to create a new balance in our biology and hormones, optimizing our mind and body, rejuvenating our physical activity, and implementing a robust approach to nutrition and supplementation, we can experience the positive health benefits we desire. Considering these efforts from a biomolecular perspective, we can expect improved epigenetic performance in our bodies over time, as our cellular turnover is complete within seven years.

The law supports those who take action and help themselves. In simpler terms, the compensation we receive reflects our effort and contributions. This basic representation of the law emphasizes the necessity of action and strength on our part. It is reminiscent of the Law of Karma, which states that we will reap what we sow.

The Bible teaches the same principle: *"Whatever a man sows, that he will also reap."* (Galatians 6:7 KJV)

In other words, we are bound by the thoughts and beliefs we hold dear, and understanding their impact and how to utilize them is the key to achieving optimal health freedom. Many of us are burdened by detrimental beliefs developed over the years, influenced by trusted advisors in health matters such as parents, physicians, friends, pharmacists, colleagues, acquaintances, and unreliable online sources. These limiting beliefs have been reinforced through repetition, leading to the health outcomes we currently experience. Whether we like it or not, we are being compensated based on the health karma we have generated for ourselves, impacting us and those around us. That is why our Medical Mastermind must consist of like-minded professionals who share the harmonious goal of achieving optimal health outcomes.

Our health reflects our beliefs and the vision we hold for our well-being. Therefore, it is crucial to intervene in the mind and limiting beliefs, as they play a significant role in shaping our health outcomes. We can maintain vibrant health for years if we hold positive beliefs about our health, supported by the right thoughts, actions, and habits. A prime example is individuals like Jack LaLanne and other health and fitness mentors who have demonstrated long-term well-being. They believe in optimizing metabolic and hormonal balance, nutrition, exercise, mind-body coherence, and envisioning a future of well-being rather than disease.

It is essential to cease verbalizing negative health outcomes immediately. We must consistently and deliberately make positive statements about our health, even if they may not feel or appear "real" in the moment. Avoid making statements such as "I'm always sick," "I always get the flu," "I'm going to get cancer," or "My family has diabetes, so I'm sure I'm going to get it." These statements only align us with the energy of ailments and diseases, inviting them into our lives. We must remember that our supply is abundant, and anything we ask for or demand from the universe will be provided, regardless of whether we initially perceive it as a frivolous request.

Accidents, aging, and death itself result from holding
incorrect mental pictures.
We become radiant beings beyond time, birth,
and death when we see ourselves as God sees us.

The good news is that the law always works, and our active effort to change our thoughts, actions, and beliefs regarding our health will yield results over time. The changes we experience will be the compensation for the effort we invest, much like a bodybuilder who progressively lifts heavier weights and sees the neuro-connectivity for that thought grow stronger over time.

However, there are no shortcuts in this domain. The Law of Compensation complements the Law of Cause and Effect, producing results from our actions. If we are healthy, happy, and wealthy, it is because we are being compensated for our positive efforts. Conversely, if our outcomes are negative, we receive compensation accordingly. By understanding these laws, we can move forward with the understanding that we can achieve any level of health, regardless of our starting point. All possibilities are available to us, beginning with our thoughts and images. These investments will provide us with compensation repeatedly. Becoming more aware of how we perceive our choices and make decisions related to our health actions is crucial. At times, making conscious decisions can be more challenging, but it is within our power to make positive changes.

Our intuitive responses, connected to infinite intelligence, can often guide us in making spontaneous health-related decisions without extensive research or contemplation. These intuitive impressions can be obtained through various methods, such as muscle testing or "gut feelings." A sense of well-being and a relaxed, reassuring feeling typically accompany a positive, intuitive response. Conversely, if an action harms our health, we may experience an ominous sensation, indicating that we should avoid it. It is important to be aware of subconscious decisions that may occur reflexively and potentially negatively impact our cells' epigenetic manifestations. Being present in the moment and making conscious health decisions are crucial to promoting well-being in our lives.

When we focus on seeking the good within ourselves rather than engaging in self-criticism and negative self-talk, we can evolve into individuals who genuinely love, nurture, and honor ourselves. This shift naturally reflects in our health status and overall quality of life. This mindset is critical for our optimized health for two reasons: first, it keeps us focused on our desired outcome and health perfection in the present moment, and second, it helps us avoid the stress-inducing environment created by condemnation or negative judgments about our health status or outcomes, which can adversely affect our hormonal and metabolic balance.

By channeling our mind's energy towards ideas of abundance, love, happiness, joy, and health, we can manifest these qualities in our lives. The Law of Compensation rewards us with appropriate benefits in exchange for our efforts, losses, or defects. In terms of our well-being, this can manifest as improved organ function across different areas, compensating for deficits or developing substitute behaviors to address perceived deficiencies. For example, stroke recovery often involves the compensatory development of other abilities, and some individuals who lose their sight experience improved hearing. To achieve better health, we need to sow the idea of and prepare for it by directing our thoughts and energy toward the desired outcome. It is important to be grateful for our current health foundation, as it serves as a springboard for reaching the next level of well-being.

"Success requires no explanations; failure allows no alibis."
—Napoleon Hill, Author of Think and Grow Rich

The Law of Compensation and the Law of Receiving plays a significant role in resolving health challenges, particularly for individuals recovering from adult-onset diabetes and obesity. The most profound results are achieved when patients actively engage in imaging and autosuggestion exercises (positive affirmations), which can be further enhanced by brainwave entrainment programming. I recommend incorporating these exercises into daily routines in the morning and evening, and during periods of heightened stress that may jeopardize progress or compliance.

Another reason for failure, indirectly linked to noncompliance with the Law of Compensation, is the expectation of gaining something for nothing or anticipating exceptional outcomes without putting in significant effort. It is unrealistic to expect improvement in our condition while making minimal or no contributions to our well-being.

Let's not delve extensively into the promises of pharmaceuticals, which often rely on the law of averages—positive effects for some individuals balanced with adverse side effects for an "acceptable" portion of users. Each of us has a unique genetic makeup (genome), and our health circumstances require personalized approaches for optimal results. This is the fundamental principle of precision medicine, which utilizes findings from the Human Genome Project and epigenomic medicine.

However, overcoming the misconception that ideal results can be achieved without compensatory effort solely through pharmaceuticals can be challenging. Countless long-term, complicated diabetics have experienced complete resolution of their "disease" by implementing simple lifestyle modifications and hormone optimization, allowing them to discontinue insulin therapy and oral medication. Similar success stories exist for patients dealing with hypertension and depression. Both patients and physicians are reaping the consequences of their choices and actions.

When we fail to dedicate our time, service, and effort to educate ourselves and surround ourselves with the right people, providers, and information necessary to make informed decisions about our health, we contribute nothing to be compensated for. To achieve the health success we deserve, it is essential to invest in our well-being and join a supportive community like the Medical Mastermind.

* * *

The Think and Live Longer Mind Shift Hack:
Energy In = Energy Out!

You have diligently applied the Mindset Hacks discussed in previous chapters and incorporated a gratitude journal into your routine. Well done!

Now, let's delve into the practical application of the Law of

Compensation in relation to health. Simply put, this law states that the input we invest will directly correspond to the output we receive. In other words, the energy we put in equals the energy we get out. We easily understand and apply this concept to our careers and jobs: if we do the work, we get paid; if we don't do the work, we don't get paid, or worse, we may lose our job. However, we tend to overlook this law in other areas of our lives, such as relationships and health.

You chose to read this book for a reason. Something about it resonated with you, whether it was the title, "Think and Live Longer," the cover image, or perhaps the Table of Contents. Your attraction to this book indicates that a part of you is ready for improved health and a better life. You already recognize that the effort you have put into your health is insufficient to achieve the change you want. It may feel like your efforts are not being adequately compensated. But here you are, reading and actively applying the laws discussed in the book. Congratulations! You are engaging with the Law of Compensation, and with consistent and mindful application, you will begin to see the results of your efforts. Energy in equals energy out; there is no other way.

Now, let's ask some critical questions:

- What do I want to achieve regarding my optimized health? (Review the "Visualize Your Health" Mindset Hack and optimize your mental image of successful health using the Form, Feeling, and Function process and handout.)
- Why do I want it? (Think about the fantastic things you can do, the places you will travel, and the level of energy,

vibrancy, and vitality you will experience.)
- How much energy am I willing to invest to attain it?

By answering these questions honestly, you can gain clarity and lay the foundation for achieving your desired level of health. Remember, the Law of Compensation applies, and your effort will directly impact the outcomes you achieve.

The Infinite Law of Allowance in Health

*"Love the hand that fate deals you and play it as your
own,*
for what could be more fitting?" – Marcus Aurelius

The Infinite Law of Allowance in Health holds immense significance and must be correctly harnessed and implemented in our daily lives. By using this law, we gain valuable insights into our optimal health and find peace and stress relief. This benefit is particularly useful in preventing and reducing certain diseases, such as hypertension and diabetes.

Today, I conversed with at least five patients struggling with various health challenges. "I can't seem to lose the weight I want," "I'm fighting my cancer," and "I'm determined to overcome this depression and anxiety." These are the common refrains I hear daily as I tap into the universal energy and try to clarify how to apply the Law of Allowance to patients who have yet to fully grasp the guidance offered to them through these disease processes.

When we contemplate the importance of balance in fostering creativity and applying it to our health, we realize that aligning ourselves harmoniously with the universal laws is crucial for achieving our desired state of empowered health. In other words, when we relax and allow harmonious alignment to guide us, we open the doors to manifest our desires. Therefore, if good health is our goal, our thoughts, beliefs, actions, and daily habits must align with that intention.

To put it simply, the law states: What we resist persists. This applies to all aspects of life, especially our health. Any issue or problem we struggle to resolve, any situation we brace ourselves against with unwavering determination, cannot be effectively addressed because our resistance perpetuates its persistence. But why does this happen?

The infinite laws are based on harmony and equilibrium. Therefore, can we truly achieve balance and equilibrium by responding to annoyances or challenges with resistance? In most cases, when two objects collide with force and momentum, the outcome is far from pleasant. This can be likened to the irresistible force paradox, which ponders the consequences when an unstoppable force encounters an immovable object. Similarly, in the realm of health, can we reduce stress on an organ system by introducing opposing stress? The answer is no.

"External things are not the problem. It's your assessment of them,
which you can erase right now." - Marcus Aurelius

Let's consider diabetes as an example. Elevated blood sugar levels are often the result of insufficient insulin or compromised insulin activity, whether due to reduced quantity or reduced effectiveness. Now, let's introduce the concept of resistance to this disease state. Resistance, in any form, is considered a new stress because it opposes achieving harmony and equilibrium. What does this lead to in our bodies and health? Any form of stress triggers a stress response, creating a reactive environment with further biochemical and hormonal imbalances that hinder insulin's function. From a metabolic and hormonal perspective, increased cortisol, epinephrine, and growth hormone levels during a stress response require significantly higher insulin levels to accomplish their tasks. "Fighting" diabetes triggers a stress response, exacerbating the imbalance and aggravating the disease.

"You become what you give your attention to... If you yourself don't choose what thoughts and Images you expose yourself to, someone else will. -Epictetus

The Infinite Law of Allowance teaches us to direct our energy toward our desired state of optimal health while accepting our current health status. By accepting and taking responsibility for our present health, we elevate our vibrational energy to align with the improved health we seek. Instead of fighting, blaming, or resisting our current undesired health, we focus on nurturing the positive aspects. A proverb illustrates this concept: a man tells his friend that he feels as if he has two wolves inside him, an evil wolf and a good wolf. When asked which wolf wins, the man replies, "The one I feed." Whenever we invest our energy in thoughts, complaints, or discussions about what we don't want (such as obesity, pain, fatigue, or lack of energy), we feed the wrong wolf. Engaging in the "fight" against our health situation depletes our resources. It is more beneficial to focus on the positive energy of aligning ourselves with the image of our optimized health.

Our focus must always be on the attributes we desire and expect to have. This is the Law of Supply and the Law of Attraction in action. Any obstacles we encounter on our journey toward optimal health result from our past thoughts, actions, and beliefs. By acknowledging this, we become less resistant to challenges and situations and create momentum for innovation. This moment of release is often followed by intuitive ideas and epiphanies that aid constructive, favorable resolutions. When we know and accept our current health as it is, we align ourselves with universal harmony, allowing universal knowledge and resources to inspire us creatively and provide timely assistance.

Regardless of the circumstances, we should not worry about finding potential solutions or dwell on existing challenges. Worry represents resistance. Instead, we should experience a sense of relaxation and comfort through the release. By choosing not to create stress in our bodies, we establish a healthier metabolic, hormonal, and immunologic environment.

How do we achieve the ideal health we envision through our exercises? By accepting ourselves and our current health without exception. It is what it is. Gratitude for our awareness, which enables us to conceptualize our current health status and the insights it offers, places us directly in the state of allowance.

I often use the metaphor of a small stream growing into a river to illustrate this process. The stream encounters various obstacles on its path to becoming a river and often changes its route to circumvent them. Initially, the small stream lacks the strength to displace even the smallest obstacles. However, as it gains power, it can overcome some obstacles. This progression not only brings the stream closer to its larger, more forceful self but also provides perspective on better pathways along the way. If the stream were to slow down and fight a larger stone or stem instead of flowing around it, it would waste energy.

Simply allowing setbacks and challenges to arise is part of the journey toward our optimized health. We should view obstacles and challenges as opportunities or blessings, as they may unknowingly present shortcuts or detours that bring us closer to our health goals. It is akin to being treated to an incredible view of fall foliage that we would have missed if not for an "annoying" detour caused by a roadblock. Bless the obstacle and move on!

> *"Whatever happens has been waiting to happen since*
> *the beginning of time. The twining strands of fate wove*
> *both of them together."*
> - Marcus Aurelius, Meditations.

With this newfound perspective, we can now embrace and

accept our current state of health. We understand that no single individual or event is to blame for this situation, and we are not at fault for its manifestation. We recognize that the universe is working in our favor, and everything is unfolding as it should. From this standpoint, we see our circumstances as an opportunity to choose peaceful, harmonious, creative, and decisive responses.

Ultimately, this attitude of allowance cultivates gratitude and brings forth elevated vibrational energy accompanied by joy. These qualities facilitate improved health. Just like a small stream growing into a mighty river, the momentum toward an empowered state of well-being continues to build.

* * *

The Think and Live Longer Mind Shift Hack:
Learning the Art of Allowance

Living in a state of allowance can be challenging for many people, especially when it comes to their health. The concept may seem simple, but it goes against our instincts. A scene from the movie, "The Sorcerer's Stone," illustrates this well. Harry, Ron, and Hermione are trapped in "Devil's Snare" vines while searching for the stone. Their natural reaction is to struggle and fight against the vines. However, Hermione remembers resisting, which worsens the situation, and advises her friends to stop moving. This is a clear example of resistance blocking what they want: survival.

Another example is the Chinese handcuffs, where the more you struggle, the tighter the hold becomes. These examples demonstrate the importance of allowance. So, how do we enter a state of allowance? It starts with recognizing when we are in a state of resistance. If we find ourselves fighting, struggling, or swimming against the current, and our efforts seem to generate more of what we don't want (such as compromised health), it's a sign that we must make a different choice.

Choosing to relax into the situation, even if it feels counterintuitive, is how we practice being in allowance. It's a conscious decision to release the struggle that no longer serves us. Using mantras can help in this process. Personally, I often use "All is well" or "Everything I desire is in the flow." Repeating these mantras helps me internalize them mentally, emotionally, physically, and spiritually. As I relax and shift my state of being, my reality starts to reflect a life experience that aligns with the flow.

Your Mind Shift Hack is to become aware of when you are in resistance. Awareness is crucial. Once you are aware, choose to relax into and allow whatever you are experiencing that you don't prefer. Trust that even in challenging situations, there is a purpose to serve and support you. It may be an opportunity to reveal what you don't prefer, prompting a shift in energy, attention, and focus toward what you do prefer.

Remember, *all is well.*

The Infinite Law of Forgiveness in Health

"It is in pardoning that we are pardoned." - Saint
Francis of Assisi

Do you remember Steven, the patient we discussed in Chapter 5, "The Infinite Law of Attraction in Health"? He was a forty-nine-year-old with several chronic health issues and a smoking habit of one to one-and-a-half packs daily. However, after starting his treatment with me, Steven responded well to the smoking cessation process I use in my practice.

This process involves "The Why List." First, Steven created a list of situations or triggers that made him want to smoke, such as work-related stress or socializing with friends who smoke. We called this the "triggering why" list. Second, Steven reflected on why he wanted to smoke. We referred to this as the "philosophical why," where he recognized potential negative outcomes like cancer, COPD, heart attacks, strokes, and more. Finally, Steven selected alternative activities to replace smoking for each trigger on his list. These activities were listed on the "replacement list" and included options such as chewing gum, sucking on candy, biting fingernails, chewing on a pen cap, or running. It's important to note that vaping was not considered an acceptable replacement activity.

After completing these exercises, Steven set a date to stop smoking. The plan involved gradually reducing his cigarette consumption by implementing the suggestions from the replacement list. Eventually, he was able to quit smoking completely. This process aligns with the practical application of the Infinite Law of Forgiveness in Health, which we will explore further.

The knowledge we have gained from the Human Genome Project and ongoing research on epigenetic modulations allows us to develop personalized programs for individuals. These programs consider an individual's genetic risks and unique responses to different exposures throughout their lifetime.

Many of the diseases that burden us result from our erroneous behavior. Erroneous beliefs give rise to thoughts that drive behaviors detrimental to optimal health. These behaviors can contribute to the development of aggravating diseases. Once we recognize and acknowledge these erroneous behaviors, it becomes necessary to forgive ourselves. This concept may sound puzzling, so let me explain further.

Consider how our bodies acquire diseases: A significant portion (seventy-five to ninety percent) is attributed to our exposures and lifestyles. Our inherited genetic material influences our bodies, and exposures can come from external sources such as bacteria, viruses, fungi, parasites, and toxins, as well as from internal sources primarily originating from our mental state. The effects of these exposures or insults may manifest immediately or after an unavoidable delay. Immediate manifestations include infections and acute trauma, while long-term effects can lead to permanent or temporary changes in our genetic material. The onset of symptoms may be delayed, depending on an individual's remaining reserves and the specific organ systems involved.

The body can be compared to a petri dish, similar to what scientists use to culture various organisms and body parts. Scientists can now place stem cells into solutions to generate specific cell types or organs. Like Petri dishes, our bodies are constantly exposed to various substances and environments through the bloodstream. The content of the fluids our cells are exposed to determines how our genes are expressed. Diseases can result when harmful substances or agents are distributed throughout the body. These diseases follow documented patterns and can range from unpleasant to life-threatening. The toxic exposures we face come from the external environment or are often self-created through our thought processes, leading to stressors.

Mark Twain once said, *"I have had many worries in my life; some of them were even real."* In an article titled "When Physicians Counsel About Stress: Results of National Study," Aditi Nerurkar, MD, MPH; Asaf Bitton, MD, MPH; Roger B. Davis, ScD; Russell S. Phillips, MD; and Gloria Yeh, MD, MPH share the results of their study on the correlation between stress and overall health. They found that sixty to eighty percent of primary care visits are related to stress. This suggests that internal causes of disease should be considered prevalent. Following the petri dish analogy, we can conclude that an individual's thoughts, which shape the body's internal environment, play a major role in overall health.

Numerous clinical and epidemiological studies have demonstrated the negative effects of stress on psychiatric diseases. However, cardiovascular disease, immune system function and dysfunction, and various other individual diseases can also be influenced. These findings are supported by a Journal of the American Medical Association article titled "Psychological Stress and Disease," in which psychologists from Carnegie Mellon University reviewed stress's contributions to multiple psychiatric and non-psychiatric diseases. At-risk populations have shown significant increases in the incidence, progression, and adverse outcomes of cardiovascular disease, autoimmune disease, HIV, cancer, upper respiratory tract infections, herpes viral infections, and impaired wound healing.

We need to examine the ideas and beliefs we hold, consciously or subconsciously, that hinder our perfect health and our ability to achieve it. It is necessary to let go of outdated beliefs or perceived knowledge that we constantly dwell on, consciously or subconsciously, to empower a renewed, reinforced image of vibrant well-being for the future.

How can we accomplish this? By forgiving the thoughts or beliefs that restrict our empowered image of optimal health. Clearing these ideas and beliefs may be more challenging if they have been ingrained in us by trusted individuals, including healthcare practitioners who may not be familiar with the improved outcomes achieved through integrated modalities.

In this context, forgiveness means letting go of the originating (erroneous) thought or idea and replacing it with accurate information. Unless we eliminate these limiting beliefs and thoughts, we cannot embrace new, invigorating, constructive, and healthy ones.

Solomon's words in Proverbs 28:13, "He that covers his sins [limiting beliefs, ideas, thoughts] shall not prosper: but whoever confesses [recognizes] and forsakes [corrects] them shall have mercy [be forgiven]," highlight the connection between thoughts and sin. Therefore, any erroneous thought can be considered equivalent to sin.

James Allen, in his book Byways of Blessedness, reflected on forgiveness as follows: *"The hard-hearted and unforgiving suffer most... for not only do they, by the law of attraction, draw revengeful passions from others, but their hardness of heart is a continuous source of suffering."*

Allen explains that forgiveness brings five types of blessings: love, increased communion and fellowship, a calm, peaceful mind, suppressed passion and pride, and kindness and good-will from others.

When we forgive, we are forgetting, abandoning, correcting, and relinquishing the condition (disease), thoughts (wrong ideas and concepts), or persons who prompted the wrongdoing, insult, or offense that occurred. We are replacing lousy information with good. The act of forgiveness enables us to create a higher vibrational energy of prosperity, health, happiness, and abundance. It eliminates negative, low-energy thoughts that lead to a lower-energy consciousness. Read again: lousy information will result in adverse outcomes that will create stress, malaise, disease, and, therefore, a self-perpetuating low-energy consciousness. Forgiveness enables us to advance to a stimulating, energetic, and healthy life!

Reflecting on wrongdoing often keeps us dwelling in the past or in imaginary future scenarios. These fictional, disempowering scenarios prevent us from focusing on the positive aspects of our future health goals. We drain our energy and strength by constantly revisiting the stressors and concerns in our lives. This prolonged stress response exacerbates metabolic and endocrine imbalances, leading to inflammation, high blood pressure, diabetes, insomnia, and further difficulties with memory, attitude, anxiety, depression, irritability, pain, fatigue, and chronic illness. I often use the analogy of "driving in the rear view mirror." Engaging in this activity inevitably leads to disastrous collisions and more obstacles, resulting in obvious and painful outcomes.

The practice of focused imaging plays a crucial role in establishing a powerful and effective health image, helping to overcome any potential resistance. Additionally, many individuals benefit from using biofeedback, which further strengthens the process of forgiveness and directs conscious and subconscious thoughts toward achievable positive goals for optimal health. When physicians or practitioners transition into the role of partner coach, counselor, or teacher within the patient-partner relationship, they become the catalysts for promoting forgiveness.

* * *

The Think and Live Longer Mind Shift Hack: Making the Lists

In this Mind Shift Hack, you will implement the "Why List" and "Replacement List" concepts discussed in the previous chapter. Although typically applied in Infinite Health Integrative Medicine Center's "Smoking Cessation Program," you can adapt this Mind Shift Hack to address any addiction or undesired behavior you wish to overcome, such as overeating or reducing alcohol intake. Follow these steps to implement the hack effectively:

The Triggering Why: Answer the following questions and write down your responses.

What is the reason behind my behavior?

What is my motivation?

Why am I choosing to engage in [fill in the blank]?

What are the specific triggers that prompt my behavior?

The Philosophical Why: Reflect on the following question and write down your answer.

Why am I even considering engaging in [fill in the blank] in the first place? (This step involves acknowledging potential negative outcomes associated with your behavior, such as cancer, COPD, heart attacks, strokes, etc.)

The Replacement List: Identify alternative activities to substitute for the undesired behavior. Write down your chosen activities for each trigger.

For example, you could consider chewing gum, sucking on candy, biting your fingernails, chewing on a pen cap, running, etc.

Complete these steps for each "Triggering Why" you have identified.

After completing this Mindset Hack, set a target date for yourself to discontinue the addiction or behavior. Write down the date and display it somewhere visible, where you will encounter it daily. Remember, you can achieve this goal. Stay determined and committed to your journey of change.

The Infinite Law of Sacrifice in Health

"The secret of change is to focus all of your energy not
on fighting the old,
but on building the new" -Socrates

Jane, a vibrant forty-two-year-old woman with a history of malignant melanoma, came to me seeking help for multiple issues related to obesity, weight gain, mood swings, fatigue, and poor tolerance of her oral antidepressants. She aimed to achieve a bikini body for the upcoming summer beach season.

Jane had undergone a total hysterectomy in her late thirties without hormone replacement therapy. She started taking antidepressants about six months after the surgery, coinciding with significant weight gain. She also underwent chemotherapy after her surgery for melanoma. During my evaluation, I discovered that her thyroid function was suboptimal and required attention.

As part of my initial assessment, I asked Jane to keep a two-week nutritional diary to understand her dietary habits.

Her diary revealed a typical diet for residents of southern Louisiana, including rice with gravy, gumbo, and boudin (a type of Cajun sausage). Jane's beverage of choice was Dr. Pepper, which she consumed three to six cans of daily.

After completing her evaluations, I initiated hormonal optimization by prescribing bioidentical estradiol, progesterone, and testosterone to address hormonal imbalances. I also discussed her suboptimal thyroid function with Armour thyroid medication. We had a detailed discussion about nutrition, focusing on reducing her carbohydrate intake. Additionally, we addressed an exercise plan and her participation in our mind-body program.

Initially, Jane responded well to the hormonal and nutritional changes, and we were able to reduce and eventually discontinue her antidepressant medication gradually. However, she hit a plateau in her fitness progress despite claiming to follow the prescribed nutritional and exercise guidelines.

Follow-up laboratory tests showed significant improvement compared with her initial results, but her A1C indicated persistently high average blood glucose levels. I asked Jane to keep another two-week nutrition diary. When she returned, I discovered she still consumed multiple cans of Dr. Pepper daily. At this point, I suggested she consult another specialist who better aligns with her goals, especially for achieving her desired bikini-season physique. This conversation served as a turning point for Jane. She sacrificed her Dr. Pepper habit, which reignited her weight loss journey and improved her glycemic control, leading to a normalized A1C.

The Infinite Law of Sacrifice holds different meanings for each individual, but the underlying principle is that to achieve something, we must sacrifice something else. These sacrifices are not insignificant, but they are made with the expectation of greater benefits. In the context of our health, it means recognizing that for every improvement in our well-being, we must be willing to give up less desirable health behaviors or habits.

This law of sacrifice complements the Laws of Receiving and Compensation. The key is to anticipate and prepare for the sacrifices required, approaching them with the necessary discipline to make them happen.

By forfeiting or sacrificing a habit, we receive (are compensated with) what we truly desire in the long term. It is healthier to forfeit the characteristic or habit that we intuitively perceive needs to go than to have something unexpected befall us due to undisciplined or ignorant self-neglect. This self-neglect may be true from many perspectives as we live and consume our extraordinary reserve.

Each organ system in our body responds differently to beneficial and detrimental influences from our internal and external environments. These influences trigger a cascade of epigenetic changes that can positively or negatively affect our reserves, resulting in consumption, enhancement, or no change.

In Matthew 7:14, Jesus states, "*Straight is the gate, and narrow is the way, which leadeth unto life, and few there be that find it*" (KJV). From a health standpoint, the Infinite Law of Sacrifice can be understood as follows: Life's abundant wealth is available to us, but cannot be attained through chance or an ignorant lifestyle devoid of healthy behaviors. Achieving our desired goals and an empowered life requires a disciplined and informed approach tailored to each individual.

One of the paradoxes of Truth is that we gain by letting go and lose by clinging. Every step toward virtue requires relinquishing some vice, and every progression in holiness involves sacrificing selfish pleasures and shedding self-assertive errors.

In pursuing optimal health, the discipline we must embrace often requires sacrifice and letting go to achieve physical and mental well-being. Conversely, the lack of discipline in eliminating undesirable behaviors (which likely contributes to the progression and persistence of such epigenetic activity) hinders our progress. For example, in cases of obesity and Type 2 diabetes, one should sacrifice the consumption of carbohydrates or quit smoking in cases of chronic bronchitis.

Those elements in our lives that are beneficial and serve us are generally not the ones that will need to be eliminated (sacrificed), obviously. Those that are detrimental by virtue of their unconscious and/or uninformed nature will need to be sacrificed to benefit our health. Additionally, our investment (the sacrifice we make) and the effort of our giving (the Infinite Law of Receiving) create the superior value of the empowered outcome we desire and achieve.

These two infinite laws serve as the currency by which we determine the compensation for the health outcome we envision. If we obtain significant health benefits without making the necessary sacrifices (personal investments), it is unlikely that we will experience long-term advantages.

An example in health and wellness is trying to lose weight through medications or surgery. These weight-loss methods often have high failure rates because little or no value is placed on achieving them. Long-term studies on laparoscopic gastric banding, for instance, reveal high overall failure rates, with more than 25% experiencing failure within 18 months and only 40% achieving long-term weight loss success (i.e., a 60% failure rate at ten years) with this popular procedure.

Oral weight loss medications often result in rebound obesity and can lead to hypertension and long-term heart damage.

Another example pertains to our suboptimal nutritional lifestyle. It is beneficial to sacrifice high-glycemic-index carbohydrates, which rapidly raise blood sugar levels. Elevated blood glucose levels contribute to the development of advanced glycation end products (AGEs), which bind to proteins within our cells. AGEs generate free radicals that cause oxidative damage to our cells' metabolism. By reducing our reliance on carbohydrate-rich diets and adopting more thoughtful, beneficial nutritional practices, we can improve our health and enhance our potential for a longer, healthier life.

Adhering to a disciplined approach in any area of health optimization ultimately yields positive results. Initially, the sacrifices required to change behavioral habits may seem challenging, but they align with the Infinite Law of Receiving. Any temporary suffering from forfeiting unhealthy habits brings immeasurable long-term benefits. Many individuals following a low-carbohydrate nutritional program to eliminate diabetes can attest to this truth. By reducing carbohydrate intake to the necessary minimum and avoiding excessive consumption, they have often eliminated the need for expensive oral and injected medications. Moreover, they experience resolution of the degenerative complications associated with elevated blood sugar levels, such as nerve damage, vascular disease, kidney failure, medication side effects, pain, and depression. We have witnessed a significant reduction in adult-onset diabetes through the disciplined adoption of a low-carbohydrate nutritional approach.

The losses we incur through sacrifice, discipline, prioritization, and behavioral modifications are replaced by vastly improved health outcomes and an enduring sense of well-being that extends beyond the temporary gratification of indulging in unhealthy treats.

We employ techniques such as replacing perceived pleasures with healthy alternatives to help with the challenging transition. Additionally, we use biofeedback training to reduce anxiety and compulsive behaviors during this period of change.

The initial weeks of the Think and Live Longer program present exhilarating challenges. It is a time for creativity and honest introspection.

* * *

The Think and Live Longer Mind Shift Hack: Creating Space

When we intentionally create an environment that aligns with our desires, we send a signal that we are ready to invite new experiences, people, or things into our lives. For instance, if we seek a new romantic partner, we can make. room for them by sleeping on one side of the bed in the middle. Similarly, if we desire a new wardrobe, we can declutter by removing clothes and accessories that no longer fit or reflect our style. These actions, in accordance with the Law of Sacrifice, accelerate our progress toward our goals.

The same approach can be applied to our pursuit of optimized health. In the upcoming days, actively engage with the infinite Law of Sacrifice by decluttering your space and creating room for empowered health. Here's a simple guide to get you started, but feel free to go beyond these suggestions as you feel guided to do so:

Kitchen Space Clearing:

Refrigerator: Clear out the refrigerator, wipe down the shelves, and discard anything that has expired or no longer aligns with your health goals.

Pantry: Apply the same approach to your pantry, removing expired items. Additionally, eliminate white flour, white sugar, white potatoes, and white rice, as they do not support your health goals. Remember, this step is about creating space and letting go of what no longer serves you.

Wardrobe Space Clearing: Tackle your closet: Take out every item from your closet. Consider donating anything you haven't worn in over a year or don't absolutely love. Discard items that no longer fit you properly. Exceptions can be made for one article of clothing that is in your ideal size and holds sentimental value. Keep it visible as a source of inspiration and motivation for your health goals.

Clearing Other Spaces: Extend the space-clearing process to every room in your house, office, car, and even to your relationships. By removing clutter and letting go of what no longer serves you, you create space for new, positive energy to flow into your life.

Remember, this process is about actively participating in the Law of Sacrifice and making room for the optimized, empowered health you desire. Embrace this opportunity to declutter and create a supportive environment for your well-being.

The Infinite Law of Obedience in Health

"When I let go of what I am, I become what I might be.
When I let go of what I have, I receive what I need."
—Lao Tzu

As I approached the final chapter, I carefully reviewed several example cases to choose the best illustration of the concept I wanted to convey. This case needed to showcase the effective application of all the universal laws and serve as a foundation for your experiential understanding of these laws.

Many of the cases I examined exemplified different aspects of the laws and their practical implementation. However, as I delved deeper, I realized that many of my successful patients had experienced multiple setbacks or deviations during their journey toward health optimization. Their unwavering determination and resolve sustained their efforts and ultimately led to their success. Whether it was their intuition or their recognition of the need to implement each law, their commitment and discipline, and their fluency in applying these universal laws to their personal challenges were key factors in achieving positive outcomes.

Gaining a clear understanding of the practical nature of these laws by accepting and internalizing them is crucial for empowerment. This internalization enables us to direct our thoughts and facilitates personal growth. The level of personal involvement and participation in the exercises and mindset hacks of the Think and Live Longer program is a reliable indicator of discipline and resolve. Those who successfully embraced the program's demands were the ones who achieved success in their health journey.

"It always seems impossible until it's done." - Nelson Mandela

"To the mind that is still, the whole universe surrenders." - Lao Tzu, Tao Te Ching

Although we are each given the template of our potential future health by our parents via their shared genomic gift, are we fated to experience the same outcomes they did? We most often answer this question in the affirmative. In reality, however, this is not the case; we consciously optimize the information provided to our epigenetic infrastructure, which each of our cells contains.

By providing better information to our epigenetic pathways, we create improved intracellular environments that enhance the expression of our individual DNA sets. This leads to the realization of optimized health patterns rather than merely accepting the genetic path of our parents and ancestors.

If we want to benefit from the governance established by these laws, we must obey them. More than simply understanding the laws is required; their true value lies in adhering to them. The power and benefits lie in our submission to these laws, which requires resolve and commitment.

> It is better to conquer yourself than to win a
> thousand battles.
> Then the victory is yours. —*Buddha*

Any criminal may possess knowledge of the law, but the true benefit of that knowledge is only obtained through the force required to adhere to it—the intention to comply with the law. Through this adherence, we establish ongoing harmony with the ideals and boundaries set by the law, ultimately benefiting ourselves.

From a practical standpoint, adherence involves recognizing the occasions and parameters that necessitate obedience and thoughtfully applying the universal laws discussed in the preceding chapters. To activate our epigenetic infrastructure and unlock the potential of our genetic gifts, we must discover the practicality and thoughtfulness inherent in these laws. Only then can we obey the laws and align our pursuit of health with the health images we have created based on our inner beliefs.

In a spiritual sense, disobedience of the law is considered a sin and is met with punishment proportional to the degree of disobedience. This punishment is a natural consequence of our errant behavior. In the context of health, the penalty typically manifests as illness or chronic disease, exacerbating the consequences of our disobedience.

For instance, inadequate sleep compromises various bodily functions, leading to epigenetic alterations that affect metabolism, inflammation, immunity, and stress responses. Such alterations may contribute to cardiovascular disease, obesity, and cognitive decline observed in sleep-deprived individuals.

Disobeying different laws results in different penalties, and the suffering endured from each "sin" can offer insights into the law violated. In practical terms, we often recognize our failures in hindsight. However, we should not despair, as our failures are valuable teachers that can guide us toward success. For example, disregarding the Law of Allowance will likely worsen existing chronic health issues. Fighting or resisting a problem, such as diabetes, triggers a stress response that elevates cortisol, adrenaline, and growth hormone levels, which impede insulin activity and worsen blood sugar levels.

The more resistant we are to our challenges, the more stress responses we experience, in accordance with the Law of Allowance and our disobedience of it.

To achieve consistent health, we must strongly desire the outcomes we want. This aligns with the Law of Attraction and the Law of Supply, where desire, intent, and expectation play vital roles. The imaging exercises this book suggests help maintain focus and intent on the desired outcomes.

Desire and expect remarkable health, especially during the imaging exercises. Worrying, adopting a scarcity mindset, affirming negative outcomes, and doubting an optimized health outcome are all obstacles that limit our ability to attain dynamic, empowered health. Doubt, in particular, hinders and stifles our desired health. Remember, we must believe before we see (Law of Supply). Hence, it is crucial to maintain a Medical Mastermind composed of supportive individuals who reinforce and motivate our well-founded beliefs, serving as catalysts in achieving our successful health image goals. This is especially important for those with multiple problems for which our physicians have given pessimistic prognoses.

When our thoughts are consumed by chaotic health outcomes, and we constantly focus on detrimental scenarios, we are not abiding by the Law of Thinking. Specifically, our thinking needs to consistently envision our idealized health images in alignment with the Law of Supply. Understanding and obeying these laws empowers us to actively create optimized, empowered health based on the positive images we hold in our minds. Disregarding these laws leads to a perception of randomness in our health outcomes, subjecting us to various imagined illnesses. It's like being adrift at sea in a rudderless skiff, passively awaiting the next wave to engulf us.

Fortunately, any adverse outcomes can be traced back to our disobedient mindset, allowing us to forgive and correct it. This ability to track our mindset lets us realize that we are never victims of random health states.

Delays in achieving desired health outcomes or obtaining alternative results often indicate a failure to obey the Law of Compensation. In such cases, we should examine the methods employed as the root cause of failure, as the corrective measures chosen may lead to even better outcomes than initially anticipated.

Understanding these laws helps us identify paths of failure and gain perspective on improvements that can be utilized to achieve optimized recovery and convalescence. Most of these paths are not visible when we experience our failures or successes.

These laws are at play in every decision, thought, and action we take, whether we are aware of it or not. Knowing and obeying them is collectively beneficial, giving us an advantage over chance and hazard. By habitual application, we seize control of the elements that contribute to success in our lives, transforming from mere co-conspirators of perceived randomness into creators of our health. Ultimately, this guidance empowers us to take charge of our health and well-being in a manner that ensures success.

Thought (Law of Thinking) and expectation (Law of Supply and Law of Attraction) of extraordinary health and well-being manifest precisely that through adherence (Law of Receiving and Law of Increase) to the envisioned image. As we embrace this newfound obedient behavior (Law of Forgiveness), the health we obtain (Law of Compensation) replaces the issues created (Law of Sacrifice) by our historically disobedient behaviors. By consistently applying these laws, our new behaviors allow (Law of Allowance) the laws to work in our favor.

Your Invitation

Redefine What Aging Means — Join the Infinite Health Movement

You've now seen what's possible when the power of the mind aligns with the science of health optimization. The next step is living it.

At **Infinite Health Integrative Medicine Center**, we help people across the nation turn possibility into proof. Using our proprietary Think and Live Longer Mind-Body Connection Coaching and 4-Pillar Health Optimization Framework, plus Regenerative Medicine therapies, our clients are redefining what aging means — increasing energy, reversing biological age, regaining focus, and experiencing true vitality from the inside out.

Now, it's your turn.

✧ **Join Our Private Skool Community**

Connect with others who are optimizing their health and longevity, gain access to exclusive insights from Trip Goolsby, MD and LeNae Goolsby, and stay inspired with real-world success stories and tools to keep you on track.

🖥 Schedule Your $99 Introductory Consultation

In this personalized call, you'll discover exactly how Infinite Health can help you optimize your health, balance your hormones, and age in reverse — no matter where you live.

Spots for new patient consultations are limited each month, and our community continues to grow rapidly. If you've been waiting for a sign, this is it.

Your body is designed to thrive. Your mind holds the key. Take the next step toward *living younger, longer.*

☞ Visit **YourInfiniteHealth.com** or email **info@YourInfiniteHealth.com** to join our Skool community and schedule your $99 introductory call today.

Infinite Health Integrative Medicine Center
  We are redefining aging.

Check Out These Other Books by the Authors

Podcast: Your Infinite Health

* * *

Empowered Medicine

Success in the New Economy

Seven Sundays to Sweet Inner Serenity: How to Cultivate the Calm Even in the Midst of Chaos

Empower Your Life: Discover your strengths, release your fears, and follow your heart.

Woke: A-ha's, awakenings, & illuminations on the path of conscious living and enlightenment

7-Figure Healthy Habits - How healthy habits create success

Radiant Resilience

The Think & Live Longer 14-Day Gratitude Journal

DAY 1

Whoever has gratitude for their health and their body will be given more,
and will have an abundance of health to their body.
—Rhonda Byrne, Author of The Magic

I am so thankful and grateful for: _______________________________
Because ____
____

I am so thankful and grateful for: _______________________________
Because ____
____

I am so thankful and grateful for: _______________________________
Because ____
____

I am so thankful and grateful for: _______________________________
Because ____
____

I am so thankful and grateful for: _______________________________
Because ____
____

I am so thankful and grateful for: _______________________________
Because ____
____

DAY 1

I am so thankful and grateful for: ____________________________
Because ____
____

I am so thankful and grateful for: ____________________________
Because ____
____

I am so thankful and grateful for: ____________________________
Because ____
____

I am so thankful and grateful for: ____________________________
Because ____
____

* * *

DAY 2

"Natural forces within us are the true healers." —Hippocrates

I am so thankful and grateful for: ______________________________
Because ____
____

I am so thankful and grateful for: ______________________________
Because ____
____

I am so thankful and grateful for: ______________________________
Because ____
____

I am so thankful and grateful for: ______________________________
Because ____
____

I am so thankful and grateful for: ______________________________
Because ____
____

I am so thankful and grateful for: ______________________________
Because ____
____

* * *

DAY 2

I am so thankful and grateful for: _______________________________
Because ____
____

I am so thankful and grateful for: _______________________________
Because ____
____

I am so thankful and grateful for: _______________________________
Because ____
____

I am so thankful and grateful for: _______________________________
Because ____
____

* * *

DAY 3

"The world is full of magical things waiting for our wits to grow sharper." —Eden Phillpotts

I am so thankful and grateful for: _______________________________
Because ____
____

I am so thankful and grateful for: _______________________________
Because ____
____

I am so thankful and grateful for: _______________________________
Because ____
____

I am so thankful and grateful for: _______________________________
Because ____
____

I am so thankful and grateful for: _______________________________
Because ____
____

I am so thankful and grateful for: _______________________________
Because ____
____

DAY 3

I am so thankful and grateful for: ___________________________
Because ____
____

I am so thankful and grateful for: ___________________________
Because ____
____

I am so thankful and grateful for: ___________________________
Because ____
____

I am so thankful and grateful for: ___________________________
Because ____
____

* * *

DAY 4

"A hundred times every day I remind myself that my inner and outer life depends on the labors of other men, living and dead, and that I must exert myself in order to give the same measure as I have received and am still receiving." —Albert Einstein

I am so thankful and grateful for: _______________________________
Because ____
____

I am so thankful and grateful for: _______________________________
Because ____
____

I am so thankful and grateful for: _______________________________
Because ____
____

I am so thankful and grateful for: _______________________________
Because ____
____

I am so thankful and grateful for: _______________________________
Because ____
____

I am so thankful and grateful for: _______________________________
Because ____
____

DAY 4

I am so thankful and grateful for: _______________________________
Because ____
____

I am so thankful and grateful for: _______________________________
Because ____
____

I am so thankful and grateful for: _______________________________
Because ____
____

I am so thankful and grateful for: _______________________________
Because ____
____

* * *

DAY 5

*"God gave you a gift of 86,400 seconds today.
Have you used one to say 'thank you?'" —William Ward*

I am so thankful and grateful for: _________________________________
Because ____
____

I am so thankful and grateful for: _________________________________
Because ____
____

I am so thankful and grateful for: _________________________________
Because ____
____

I am so thankful and grateful for: _________________________________
Because ____
____

I am so thankful and grateful for: _________________________________
Because ____
____

I am so thankful and grateful for: _________________________________
Because ____
____

DAY 5

I am so thankful and grateful for: ___________________________
Because ____
____

I am so thankful and grateful for: ___________________________
Because ____
____

I am so thankful and grateful for: ___________________________
Because ____
____

I am so thankful and grateful for: ___________________________
Because ____
____

* * *

DAY 6

"Gratitude is the memory of the heart." —Jean-Baptiste Massieu

I am so thankful and grateful for: _______________________
Because _______________________________________
____

I am so thankful and grateful for: _______________________
Because _______________________________________
____

I am so thankful and grateful for: _______________________
Because _______________________________________
____

I am so thankful and grateful for: _______________________
Because _______________________________________
____

I am so thankful and grateful for: _______________________
Because _______________________________________
____

I am so thankful and grateful for: _______________________
Because _______________________________________
____

DAY 6

I am so thankful and grateful for: ______________________________
Because ____
____

I am so thankful and grateful for: ______________________________
Because ____
____

I am so thankful and grateful for: ______________________________
Because ____
____

I am so thankful and grateful for: ______________________________
Because ____
____

* * *

DAY 7

"You say grace before meals. All right. But I say grace before the concert and the opera, and grace before the play and pantomime, and grace before I open a book, and grace before sketching, painting, swimming, fencing, boxing, walking, playing, dancing, and grace before I dip the pen in the ink."
—*G. K. Chesterton*

I am so thankful and grateful for: _______________________
Because ____

____

I am so thankful and grateful for: _______________________
Because ____

____

I am so thankful and grateful for: _______________________
Because ____

____

I am so thankful and grateful for: _______________________
Because ____

____

I am so thankful and grateful for: _______________________
Because ____

____

I am so thankful and grateful for: _______________________
Because ____

____

DAY 7

I am so thankful and grateful for: _______________________________
Because ____
____

I am so thankful and grateful for: _______________________________
Because ____
____

I am so thankful and grateful for: _______________________________
Because ____
____

I am so thankful and grateful for: _______________________________
Because ____
____

* * *

DAY 8

"People who wait for a magic wand fail to see that they are the magic wand."
—Thomas Leonard

I am so thankful and grateful for: _______________________________
Because ____
____

I am so thankful and grateful for: _______________________________
Because ____
____

I am so thankful and grateful for: _______________________________
Because ____
____

I am so thankful and grateful for: _______________________________
Because ____
____

I am so thankful and grateful for: _______________________________
Because ____
____

I am so thankful and grateful for: _______________________________
Because ____
____

DAY 8

I am so thankful and grateful for: _________________________________
Because ____
____

I am so thankful and grateful for: _________________________________
Because ____
____

I am so thankful and grateful for: _________________________________
Because ____
____

I am so thankful and grateful for: _________________________________
Because ____
____

* * *

DAY 9

"Turn your wounds into wisdom." —Oprah Winfrey

I am so thankful and grateful for: _______________________
Because ____
____

I am so thankful and grateful for: _______________________
Because ____
____

I am so thankful and grateful for: _______________________
Because ____
____

I am so thankful and grateful for: _______________________
Because ____
____

I am so thankful and grateful for: _______________________
Because ____
____

I am so thankful and grateful for: _______________________
Because ____
____

DAY 9

I am so thankful and grateful for: ________________________________
Because ____
____

I am so thankful and grateful for: ________________________________
Because ____
____

I am so thankful and grateful for: ________________________________
Because ____
____

I am so thankful and grateful for: ________________________________
Because ____
____

* * *

DAY 10

To speak gratitude is courteous and pleasant, to enact gratitude is generous and noble, but to live gratitude is to touch Heaven. —Johannes A. Gaertner

I am so thankful and grateful for: ______________________________
Because ______________________________
____

I am so thankful and grateful for: ______________________________
Because ______________________________
____

I am so thankful and grateful for: ______________________________
Because ______________________________
____

I am so thankful and grateful for: ______________________________
Because ______________________________
____

I am so thankful and grateful for: ______________________________
Because ______________________________
____

I am so thankful and grateful for: ______________________________
Because ______________________________
____

* * *

DAY 10

I am so thankful and grateful for: _______________________________
Because ____
____

I am so thankful and grateful for: _______________________________
Because ____
____

I am so thankful and grateful for: _______________________________
Because ____
____

I am so thankful and grateful for: _______________________________
Because ____
____

* * *

DAY 11

"We showed him (i.e. man) the way: whether he be grateful or ungrateful (rests on his will). —Unknown

I am so thankful and grateful for: _______________________________
Because ____
____

I am so thankful and grateful for: _______________________________
Because ____
____

I am so thankful and grateful for: _______________________________
Because ____
____

I am so thankful and grateful for: _______________________________
Because ____
____

I am so thankful and grateful for: _______________________________
Because ____
____

I am so thankful and grateful for: _______________________________
Because ____
____

DAY 11

I am so thankful and grateful for: ______________________________
Because ____
____

I am so thankful and grateful for: ______________________________
Because ____
____

I am so thankful and grateful for: ______________________________
Because ____
____

I am so thankful and grateful for: ______________________________
Because ____
____

* * *

DAY 12

"When you arise in the morning, give thanks for the morning light, for your life and strength. Give thanks for your food and the joy of living. If you see no reason for giving thanks, the fault lies within yourself."
—Tecumseh

I am so thankful and grateful for: _______________________________
Because ____
____

I am so thankful and grateful for: _______________________________
Because ____
____

I am so thankful and grateful for: _______________________________
Because ____
____

I am so thankful and grateful for: _______________________________
Because ____
____

I am so thankful and grateful for: _______________________________
Because ____
____

I am so thankful and grateful for: _______________________________
Because ____
____

DAY 12

I am so thankful and grateful for: ____________________________
Because ____
____

I am so thankful and grateful for: ____________________________
Because ____
____

I am so thankful and grateful for: ____________________________
Because ____
____

I am so thankful and grateful for: ____________________________
Because ____
____

* * *

DAY 13

"As we express gratitude, we must never forget that the highest appreciation is not to utter words, but to live by them."—John F. Kennedy

I am so thankful and grateful for: ________________________________
Because ____
____

I am so thankful and grateful for: ________________________________
Because ____
____

I am so thankful and grateful for: ________________________________
Because ____
____

I am so thankful and grateful for: ________________________________
Because ____
____

I am so thankful and grateful for: ________________________________
Because ____
____

I am so thankful and grateful for: ________________________________
Because ____
____

DAY 13

I am so thankful and grateful for: _______________________
Because ____
____

I am so thankful and grateful for: _______________________
Because ____
____

I am so thankful and grateful for: _______________________
Because ____
____

I am so thankful and grateful for: _______________________
Because ____
____

DAY 14

"When I started counting my blessings, my whole life turned around."
—*Willie Nelson*

I am so thankful and grateful for: _______________________________
Because ____
____

I am so thankful and grateful for: _______________________________
Because ____
____

I am so thankful and grateful for: _______________________________
Because ____
____

I am so thankful and grateful for: _______________________________
Because ____
____

I am so thankful and grateful for: _______________________________
Because ____
____

I am so thankful and grateful for: _______________________________
Because ____
____

DAY 14

I am so thankful and grateful for: ____________________________
Because ____
____

I am so thankful and grateful for: ____________________________
Because ____
____

I am so thankful and grateful for: ____________________________
Because ____
____

I am so thankful and grateful for: ____________________________
Because ____
____

* * *

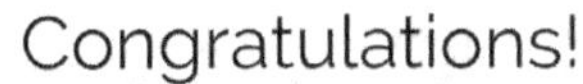

Congratulations!

You have completed the Fourteen-Day Think and Live Longer Gratitude Journal! But don't stop here!

Keep it up every day until it becomes your habit, and you will begin to see more and more infinite health flow to you!

References

[1] Hum Genet. 2006 Apr;119(3):312-21. Epub 2006 Feb 4.

* All patients' names have been changed to protect their privacy; however, in every case, I have personally been involved.

[2] Nerurkar, A., Bitton, A., Davis, R. B., Phillips, R. S., & Yeh, G. (2013). When physicians counsel about stress: results of a national study. *JAMA internal medicine, 173*(1), 76-7.

[3] Cohen S, Janicki-Deverts D, Miller GE. Psychological Stress and Disease. *JAMA.* 2007;298(14):1685–1687. doi:10.1001/jama.298.14.1685

Braden, Gregg, The Spontaneous Healing of Belief, Hay House, 2008.

Canfield, Jack, The Success Principles, Harper Collins, 2004.

Chopra, Deepak, The Seven Spiritual Laws of Success, Amber-Allen Publishing and New World Library, 1994.

Cohen S., Janicki-Deverts D., Miller, G. E., "Psychological Stress and Disease." JAMA.2007:298(14):1685–1687. doi:10.1001/jama.298.14.1685.

DeMaria, Eric J. MD; Sugerman, Harvey J. MD; Meador, Jill G. RN, BSN; Doty, James M. MD; Kellum, John M. MD; Wolfe, Luke MS; Szucs, Richard A. MD; Turner, Mary Ann MD. "High Failure Rate After Laparoscopic Adjustable Silicone Gastric Banding for Treatment of Morbid Obesity." Annals of Surgery: June 2001 Vol. 233 - Issue 6 - pp 809–818

The emperor's new drugs: An analysis of antidepressant medication data submitted to the U.S. Food and Drug Administration.

http://www.emersoncentral.com/compensation.htm

http://www.emersoncentral.com/spirituallaws.htm

http://www.goodreads.com/quotes/201777-i-ve-had-a-lot-of-worries-in-my-life-most

http://www.goodreads.com/quotes/374489-the-greatest-revolution-of-our-generation-is-thediscovery-that

http://science.sciencemag.org/content/291/5507/1304.full

Kirsch, Irving; Moore, Thomas J.; Scoboria, Alan; Nicholls, Sarah S. Prevention & Treatment, Vol 5(1), Jul 2002, No Pagination Specified Article 23.http://dx.doi.org/10.1037/1522-3736.5.1.523a

Medawar, P., The Limits of Science pg 98 (New York Harper and Row) 1984 Taken from Wiki quote at https://en.wikiquote.org/wiki/Peter Medawar

Miller, F. G., "William James, Faith, and the Placebo Effect," Perspectives in Biology and Medicine, Vol. 48 no. 2 Spring 2005, pp 273–281.

Möller-Levet, Carla S., Archer, Simon N., Bucca, Giselda, Laing, Emma E., Slak, Ana, Kabiljo, Renata, Lo, June C. Y., Santhi, Nayantara, von Schantz, Malcolm, Smith, Colin P., and Dijk, Derk-Jan. "Effects of insufficient sleep on circadian rhythmicity and expression amplitude of the human blood transcriptome." PNAS 2013 110 (12) E1132-E1141; published ahead of print February 25, 2013,doi:10.1073/pnas.1217154110

Nerurkar A, Bitton A, Davis RB, Phillips RS, Yeh G. "When Physicians Counsel About Stress: Results of a National Study." JAMA Intern Med. 2013;173(1):76–77. doi:10.1001/2013.jamainternmed.480

Suter, M., Calmes, J.M., Paroz, A. et. al. "A 10-year Experience with Laparoscopic Gastric Banding for Morbid Obesity: High Long-Term Complication and Failure Rates." OBES SURG (2006) 16: 829. Doi: 10.1381/096089206777822359

Hjelmborg JB, Iachine I, SkyXhe A, et al. Genetic influence on human lifespan and longevity. *Human Genetics.* 2006;119(3):312–321

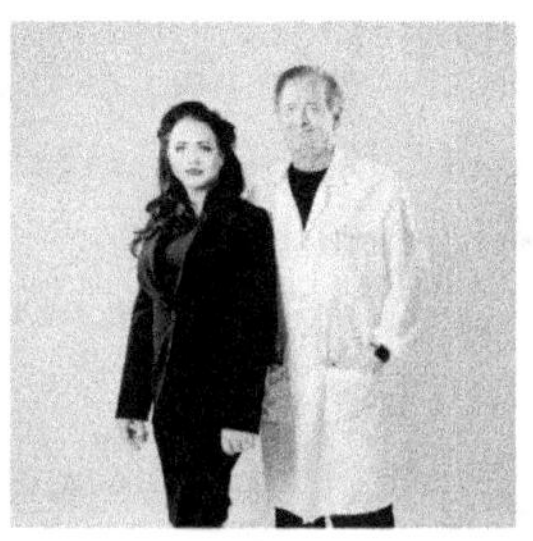

About the Author

LeNae and Trip Goolsby, MD are the founders of Infinite Health Integrative Medicine Center, a precision-medicine practice with a niche focus on health optimization, age reversal, and regenerative medicine.

LeNae and Dr. Goolsby are also best-selling authors and speakers. They have been featured experts in various internationally recognized podcasts and magazine publications, such as Brainz Magazine, MindBodyGreen.com, PsychCentral.com, Entereprener.com, and many others.

LeNae & Dr. Goolsby have also published several books, including, "Think and Live Longer," which is also their proprietary mind-body connection coaching program. "Think and Live Longer," in connection with their progressive peer-reviewed and evidence-based medical modalities, is instrumental in helping thousands of women and men transform not just their health but their lives.

LeNae and Dr. Goolsby empower people across the globe to reclaim their health power to create, and attain their personalized successful health image.

You can connect with me on:
- https://www.yourinfinitehealth.com
- https://www.facebook.com/infinitehealthimc